OATH BETRAYED

UNIVERSITY OF CALIFORNIA PRESS

Berkeley • *Los Angeles* • *London*

STEVEN H. MILES, M.D.

America's Torture Doctors

OATH
BETRAYED

Second Edition

University of California Press, one of the most distinguished university presses in the United States, enriches lives around the world by advancing scholarship in the humanities, social sciences, and natural sciences. Its activities are supported by the UC Press Foundation and by philanthropic contributions from individuals and institutions. For more information, visit www.ucpress.edu.

University of California Press
Berkeley and Los Angeles, California

Previously published in 2006 by Random House.

Library of Congress Cataloging-in-Publication Data

Miles, Steven H.
     Oath betrayed : America's torture doctors / Steven H. Miles—2nd ed.
        p.   cm.
     Includes bibliographical references and index.
     ISBN 978-0-520-25968-3 (pbk. : alk. paper)
     1. Prisoners of war—Medical care—Moral and ethical aspects.   2. Medical personnel—Professional ethics—United States.   3. Medicine, Military—Moral and ethical aspects.
4. Torture—Moral and ethical aspects.   5. Prisoners of war—Abuse of—Iraq.   6. Prisoners of war—Abuse of—Afghanistan.   7. Prisoners of war—Abuse of—Cuba.   8. War on Terrorism, 2001—Moral and ethical aspects.   9. Abu Ghraib Prison   10. Guantánamo Bay Naval Base (Cuba).   I. Title.

R725.5.M55   2009
174.2'9698023—dc22   2008049546

Manufactured in the United States of America

18   17   16   15   14   13   12   11   10   09
10   9   8   7   6   5   4   3   2   1

This book is printed on Natures Book, which contains 30% post-consumer waste and meets the minimum requirements of ANSI/NISO Z39.48-1992 (R 1997) (Permanence of Paper).

Book design by Simon M. Sullivan

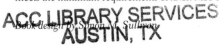

I WILL USE REGIMENS FOR THE BENEFIT OF THE ILL IN
ACCORDANCE WITH MY ABILITY AND MY JUDGMENT, BUT FROM
WHAT IS TO THEIR HARM OR INJUSTICE I WILL KEEP THEM.

—Hippocratic Oath, 500 B.C.

CONTENTS

INTRODUCTION TO THE SECOND EDITION

WHERE WERE THE DOCTORS AND NURSES AT ABU GHRAIB?

In May 2004, pictures of soldiers abusing prisoners at Abu Ghraib, a prison near Baghdad used by the U.S. military, shocked the world. When I saw these pictures, a simple question came to mind and became the genesis of this book. Surely the doctors at Abu Ghraib knew of these abuses. Why didn't they intervene? I was not the only person to ask this question.[1–3] Ensuing congressional and military investigations, however, have largely ignored the role that medical personnel played in abetting or passively acquiescing in the torture of prisoners. Defense Department investigations were tightly designed to confine responsibility to low-ranking frontline personnel in Iraq.

Four months after the Abu Ghraib photographs surfaced, *The Lancet*, a British medical journal, published my first effort to answer the question.[4] The evidence for medical complicity in prisoner abuses was taken from a leaked investigation by General Antonio Taguba, congressional testimony, and some media and human rights organizations' reports. The article received international attention. The Defense Department forwarded it to medical officers in Iraq.[5] An Army lieutenant colonel, Joseph Richard, gave the official rebuttal: "The Department of Defense takes strong exception to these allegations and [Miles's] wholesale indictment of the medical care rendered by U.S. personnel to prisoners and detainees. . . . [The article is based on] carefully selected media reports and excerpted Capitol Hill testimony and not firsthand investigative work or accounts."[6]

The question "Where were the doctors at Abu Ghraib?" became more troubling as it became clear that abuses like those depicted in the photographs were not limited to a "few bad apples," a few months, a problem cellblock, or even a single prison. Similar abuses had occurred for several years across an archipelago of U.S. war on terror prisons stretching from Guantánamo Bay to Iraq to Afghanistan, and through a clandestine network of CIA jails scattered across Europe, the Middle East, Asia, and North Africa. The abuses were pandemic. And so was the failure of doctors and psychologists to raise their voices to stop them.

In 2006, Random House published the first edition of this book, then called *Oath Betrayed: Torture, Medical Complicity, and the War on Terror.* That book was based on tens of thousands of pages of government documents obtained by the American Civil Liberties Union (ACLU) through a Freedom of Information Act lawsuit. In 2007, I put up an online archive of 50,000 pages of those government documents pertaining to the prison medical system. Cynthia Scott offered the Defense Department's Orwellian response, "Further dissemination of this material isn't in the spirit of the Freedom of Information Act program."[7]

It is now beyond doubt that Armed Forces physicians, psychologists, and medics were passive and active partners in the systematic neglect and abuse of war on terror prisoners. In Iraq and Afghanistan, the United States failed to provide prisoners with minimally adequate medical and public health care. Physicians and psychologists supplied interrogators with medical information to use in setting the nature and degree of physical and psychological abuse during interrogations. They monitored interrogations to devise ways to break prisoners down or to keep them alive. Military pathologists withheld death certificates and autopsy reports so as to enable the Defense Department to understate the number of prisoners who had died of torture or to wrongly claim that murdered prisoners had died of natural causes. They continue to withhold such information, including the particulars of the deaths of CIA prisoners and of at least one child and at least one woman. Medical personnel who knew of this system of torture and cruel, inhuman, and degrading treatment and punishment remained silent.

I reached these conclusions reluctantly. I wanted to believe that military medical personnel had tried to raise the alarm. I had expected to discover how doctors' complaints went unheeded or were suppressed. I did not expect and certainly did not hope to find that military health person-nel were part of a system for abusing prisoners. Although many medical personnel provided admirable treatment to prisoners, the number who ac-tively participated in abuse or who passively witnessed it was sufficient to allow a prison system that was (and is) unworthy of the United States to operate unchecked.

MEDICAL ETHICS AND TORTURE

This is a book on medical ethics. Fundamentally, it is about the profes-sional duty to promote the well-being of imprisoned patients. Numerous medical ethics codes bar clinicians from abetting torture. Medical com-plicity with torture and cruel, inhuman, and degrading treatment of pris-oners is not a "political" issue. The Abu Ghraib abuses summon the moral engagement of every clinician in military service, in civilian life, in med-ical societies, and on licensing boards to safeguard values that lie at the core of what it means to be a healer. The reputation of the profession is at stake. Its ability to speak on behalf of endangered prisoners or of colleagues who bravely resist their own torturing governments has been undermined.

This is not a book about medical ethics on the battlefield. It is about the treatment of disarmed and isolated captives. Those who excuse these abuses as simply part of the brutality of war fail to grasp the critical legal and moral difference between combat and prisons. The Geneva Conven-tions' phrase *hors de combat* (outside of combat), by which they refer to persons imprisoned during war or occupation, precisely names this dis-tinction. I disagree with those who say that abusing these prisoners of war is merely "rough justice" for terrorists. These acts contributed to the dis-integration of Iraq. They alienated our allies and multiplied our enemies. The first beheadings of American soldiers and contractors in Iraq oc-curred after the Abu Ghraib pictures were released. Since those pictures were released, no U.S. soldier captured in Iraq has been rescued, escaped, or traded back home.

This is not a comprehensive history of human rights abuses in the war on terror. It does not look at abuses by our allies or enemies. It cannot look at the abuses of persons whom the CIA secretly transported to countries such as Pakistan, Egypt, Romania, or Uzbekistan for imprisonment, torture, and interrogation. The United States continues to refuse to allow Red Cross or United Nations monitors unrestricted access to privately interview many prisoners. Tens of thousands of pages of U.S. documents about war on terror prisons, including many of the appendixes to declassified investigations, remain blacked out by judgments that seem designed to protect officials from embarrassment or prosecution rather than to protect national security. Prisons for "high value" persons, including the recently revealed Camp 7 at Guantánamo, remain cloaked.

I will not debate the legal nit-picking of the government policies that created these prisons. Every torturing government tries to paint a patina of law over its crimes. Any government can find lawyers or legislators who will renounce, suspend, or define away the world's settled opinion against torture as it is inscribed in documents such as the Geneva Conventions or the Convention Against Torture or Cruel, Inhuman or Degrading Treatment or Punishment. As the sirens of "national emergency" wail in nations committing torture, executives assume special powers, legislatures enact patriot acts, scribes revise regulations, courts excuse abuses, and those who wield the truncheons are sheltered from accountability. If law be the bedrock of civil society, it can no more undergird torture than it can support slavery or genocide.

The international laws and medical ethics codes pertaining to torture are not finicky rules like those constituting the bulk of ordinary federal and state laws. These are breathing expressions of global moral aspiration. Often, they are as eloquent as the Declaration of Independence or the preamble to the U.S. Constitution. One can hear both the world's horror at the Nazi death camps and the echoes of Franklin Roosevelt's famous Four Freedoms talk in the United Nations' 1948 Universal Declaration of Human Rights.

> Whereas recognition of the inherent dignity and of the equal and inalienable rights of all members of the human family is the foundation of freedom, justice and peace in the world,
>
> Whereas disregard and contempt for human rights have resulted in barbarous acts which have outraged the conscience of mankind, and the

advent of a world in which human beings shall enjoy *freedom of speech and belief and freedom from fear and want* [emphasis added] has been proclaimed as the highest aspiration of the common people, . . . No one shall be subjected to torture or to cruel, inhuman or degrading treatment or punishment.

Citizens of the global community should know these works. They ring with the same eloquence as "We hold these truths to be self evident. . . ." These profound and simple statements of human rights measure the magnitude of the abuse of prisoners in the war on terror. Unfortunately, they are relatively unknown. Few schools teach them. The United States stands nearly alone in refusing to ratify many of them. Each chapter of this book contains relevant excerpts from these documents so that readers may meet and, I hope, come to admire these remarkable documents.

A TIME LINE FOR MEDICAL COMPLICITY

Historians are still reconstructing the history of the policies allowing human rights abuses during the Bush administration. It is possible, however, to create a timeline showing how physicians and psychologists were drawn into the infrastructure of war on terror prisons. Vice President Richard Cheney, his chief of staff, David Addington, and Secretary of Defense Donald Rumsfeld exercised executive authority over the torture and prison policies. They shielded the emerging policies from critics at the State Department, Armed Forces JAG corps attorneys, Congress, and the public. John Yoo and Jay Bybee of the President's Office of Legal Counsel wrote the legal justifications and fundamental content for attorneys general John Ashcroft and Alberto Gonzales to endorse. Secretary of State Condoleezza Rice, the president, and others discussed and approved the harsh policies.

In 2002, Defense Department attorney Diane Beaver crafted Guantánamo's request for harsh interrogation techniques, arguing that such techniques were legally permissible "with appropriate medical monitoring."[8] Six months later, Secretary of Defense Rumsfeld proposed two clinical roles during interrogations. One, echoing Lieutenant Colonel Beaver, was to "safeguard" prisoners by providing preinterrogation clearances and intrainterrogation monitoring. The second was to use behavioral scientists to help create ways to "manipulate the detainee's emotions and weaknesses to gain his willing cooperation."[9] Behavioral Science Consultation Teams (BSCTs, or "Biscuits") were the offspring of that latter role.

From their inception, BSCTs were created to facilitate the harsh interrogations that the administration had elected to employ. Major General Geoffrey Miller defined the BSCT mission in terms of assisting in intelligence gathering.[10] BSCTs reported to military intelligence rather than to health affairs.[11] The Defense Department's deputy assistant secretary for health, Dr. David Tornberg, said there was "no doctor-patient relationship" for interrogatees.[12] In 2005, Army Surgeon General Kevin Kiley rejected the recommendation that psychiatrists or physicians not serve as BSCT members.[13] In June 2006, the Defense Department reiterated the distinction between clinicians responsible for advising interrogators and those responsible for prisoners' health.[14] (This policy supersedes the policy discussed in chapter 3 on pages 64n144 and 158n61.) Figure I.1 shows a time line of the major events in policymaking and history regarding medical personnel and prisoners.

In October 2006, the Defense Department issued a second-generation policy on BSCTs. Their mission is to "provide consultative services to support authorized law enforcement or intelligence activities, including detention and related intelligence, interrogation, and detainee debriefing operations." BSCT personnel are not to view prisoners as patients: "The Department of Defense is the identified client" to whom these clinicians owe their primary loyalty. Again, BSCTs are set within the interrogation command. Their main duty is to advise interrogators of a prisoner's "strengths and vulnerabilities" and "assist in developing and executing" interrogation plans. They are required to be experts in "learned helplessness" and to use that knowledge to advise on the application of physical and emotional stressors. In addition, they advise "on how to change the prison environment" because, as Secretary Rumsfeld put it, "interrogations should be conducted in close cooperation with the units detaining the individual." They also serve as a kind of parole advisory board on "the likelihood that a detainee will, if released, engage in terrorist, illegal,

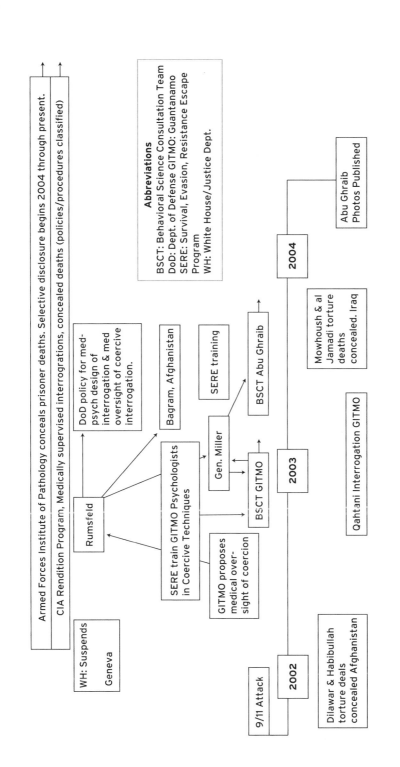

FIGURE 1.1. *Time line of command for medical complicity with human rights abuses.*

combatant, or similar activities." The current BSCT policy requires personnel to comply with applicable law even though the administration maintains that the president has the authority to suspend laws and treaties. It promotes the Geneva Conventions but pointedly does not mention the Convention Against Torture, to which the United States is also a signatory. It emphasizes that BSCT personnel must prevent and report abuse.

It is impossible to balance a primary duty of supporting coercive interrogations with the role of shortstop to catch abuse. Contradictions abound. Therapeutic personnel are not supposed to aid or interfere with interrogations but BSCT personnel can review medical records to identify vulnerabilities to exploit. BSCT personnel are not to medically clear or monitor prisoners for interrogation; those activities are considered "health care." Not surprisingly, an Army BSCT psychologist who allegedly authorized the continued mistreatment of a juvenile prisoner at Guantánamo who broke down under abusive interrogation recently refused to testify, on grounds of self-incrimination.

NEW ISSUES: DRUGS AND INTERROGATION RESEARCH

Since the first edition of *Oath Betrayed* in 2006, two disturbing new dimensions of this scandal have emerged.

There is increasing evidence that prisoners were drugged for interrogation and to facilitate the illegal kidnappings of the CIA's rendition program. The administration anticipated the use of interrogational drugs in its initial policy documents including Assistant Attorney General Jay Bybee's memo (August 1, 2002), Secretary of Defense Rumsfeld's Working Group report (April 2003), and Deputy Assistant Attorney General John Yoo's memo (March 14, 2003).[15–17] The Army surgeon general has recorded anecdotal cases of requests for such agents.[18] Media accounts report that prisoners have told their lawyers of being subjected to interrogational drugs.[19] The Senate Armed Services Committee recently released minutes of a 2002 Guantánamo interrogation policy committee meeting that discussed the potential use of "truth serum."[20] It is a breach of medical ethics for a clinician to assist in the preparation or administration of drugs for interrogation or kidnapping. The World Medical Association's Declaration of Tokyo puts it this way: "The doctor shall not provide any premises, instruments, substances or knowledge to facilitate the practice of torture or other forms of cruel, inhuman or degrading treatment or *to diminish the ability of the victim to resist such treatment*" (emphasis added).

The second emerging issue is the possibility that coerced and abusive interrogation experiments were conducted at Guantánamo. There is sufficient circumstantial evidence to warrant an investigation to determine whether Behavioral Science Consultation Teams supervised this research. Such experimentation was condemned at Nuremberg. The Geneva Convention on Prisoners of War defines such research as a war crime: "In particular, no prisoner of war may be subjected to . . . medical or scientific experiments of any kind which are not justified by the medical, dental or hospital treatment of the prisoner concerned and carried out in his interest."

The CIA and Armed Forces have long researched the utility of hypnosis, drugs, physical and emotional stress, and isolation for interrogation.[21–23] This research began after World War II with the Navy's Project CHATTER. CHATTER ended in 1953 when the CIA's Office of Scientific Intelligence launched what became a series of projects: BLUEBIRD, ARTICHOKE, MK-DELTA, MK-NAOMI, MK-ULTRA, and MK-SEARCH. The partnership between the CIA, the Armed Forces, and major universities and health professional associations continued until at least 1973.[24,25] The finding that coercion, threats, and stress were ineffective or counterproductive did not diminish interest in more studies.

Some of the findings from this research were used by behavioral scientists working at SERE (Survival, Evasion, Resistance, Escape) programs.[26–28] SERE programs serve all branches of the Armed Forces and the intelligence agencies. They prepare soldiers and intelligence personnel for the eventuality of being captured. SERE employs lectures and physical hardship, including stress positions, noise, hunger, temperature extremes, desecration of the Bible, sexual humiliation, and even waterboarding. SERE techniques were designed to simulate brutal captivity—they had not been validated for interrogation. During the war on terror, military psychologists took the SERE techniques and "reverse engineered" them for interrogation. Reverse engineering is less scientific than it sounds; it essentially consisted of picking SERE techniques to use during interrogation.[29]

The BSCTs had everything they needed to conduct research. They were an organ of military intelligence, which wanted better information. They had the authority to use and monitor abusive SERE-derived techniques to carry out interrogation. For example, SERE stress positions might be used to carry out the Army Field Manual's "fear up harsh" approach or exposure to cold could constitute "environmental manipulation." BSCT personnel were required to have scientific expertise and top secret security clearance. SERE behavioral scientists were familiar with measuring physiologic indicators including stress hormones. SERE personnel taught BSCT personnel. BSCT personnel had a captive and hidden group of prisoners whose rights of consent or refusal had been declared void. But did they take the final step? Did they create a program to research coercive interrogation?

I believe that the answer is probably yes. I discuss why in appendix 1.

THE CIVILIAN MEDICAL SECTOR'S RESPONSE

The first edition of Oath Betrayed characterized the U.S. medical community as largely silent on medical complicity in human rights abuses in war on terror prisons. A United Nations Human Rights working group sharply criticized U.S. military medicine.[30] It stated:

Health professionals in Guantánamo Bay have systematically violated widely accepted ethical standards set out in the United Nations Principles of Medical Ethics and the Declaration of Tokyo, in addition to well-established rules on medical confidentiality. Alleged violations include: (a) breaching confidentiality by sharing medical records or otherwise disclosing health information for purposes of interrogation; (b) participating in, providing advice for or being present during interrogations; and (c) being present during or engaging in non-consensual treatment, including drugging and force-feeding. In sum, reports indicate that some health professionals have been complicit in abusive treatment of detainees detrimental to their health. Such unethical conduct violates the detainees' right to health, as well as the duties of health professionals arising from the right to health. . . . The Government of the United States should revise the United States Department of Defense Medical Program Principles to be consistent with the United Nations Principles of Medical Ethics.

U.S. medical societies did not react to this high-profile condemnation by a prestigious group. The tiny Physicians for Human Rights acts as the conscience of American medicine while the largest medical societies timidly tarry in the shadows. Health professional licensing boards and societies have declined to investigate complaints or censure health care personnel when documented allegations of human rights abuses have been presented. The California legislature has passed Resolution SJR 19, which asks state licensing agencies to inform clinicians that participating in coercive interrogation or torture as defined by the Convention Against Torture may render them subject to professional and criminal sanctions.[31]

Public controversy over medical complicity with abusive interrogations has led to some strengthening of professional ethics codes since those discussed on page 175–176 of the first edition of *Oath Betrayed*. Psychiatry and psychology societies, in particular, have distanced themselves from the position of the American Psychological Association (see appendix 2).[32–36] A few medical societies have strengthened their codes on interrogation or documentation of abuses.[37,38] Although medical societies are moving toward asserting a duty to record and report the abuse of prisoners, they are not acting to hold clinicians accountable for participating or acquiescing in this abuse.[39]

EVIDENCE

This book has a conservative method. It is grounded on gleanings from tens of thousands of pages of government documents. Media reports are used sparingly, mainly for important and attributed quotations. I did not do interviews or use briefs prepared by attorneys who represent prisoners. Such material is not secured under oath and often paraphrases stories. I have not referenced popular movies such as *Ghosts of Abu Ghraib, Standard Operating Procedure, The Road to Guantánamo, Rendition,* or *Taxi to the Dark Side,* or even an episode of the television show *Law and Order,* all of which were largely derived from material that I cite directly. I wanted to write a book whose sources could be examined. I wanted to avoid interview material that, if challenged, might evaporate in claims that words were misunderstood or taken out of context.

There is a certain durable quality to primary sources such as autopsy reports, death certificates, and prisoners' medical records, sworn testimony given by soldiers to Army investigators, or Defense Department directives, policies, and e-mails dashed off in the middle of the night. Such documents tell the story with an authority that is difficult to obtain from interviews with a few dozen people who are reluctant to speak on the record. Despite their value, I would not want to overstate the veracity of government documents. Military officials routinely gave less weight to prisoners' descriptions of being abused than to soldiers' routine denials or "I can't recalls". Defense Department investigations were chartered and performed by the same institutions whose actions are being challenged. Documents have been selectively and partially declassified. The documents disproportionately come from Iraq; a few come from Guantánamo; fewer come from Afghanistan; none come from CIA prisons.

The journalists, lawyers, and human rights advocates who have excavated the history of the war on terror prisons should not be undervalued. The *Washington Post, New York Times, Los Angeles Times, Guardian, New Yorker,* and *Time* have done solid investigative reporting. News media have released a few documents that opened the door to requests for further documents. Many good books on human rights abuses in the war on terror prisons have been written. Some of the most illuminating are *Torture and Truth: America, Abu Ghraib, and the War on Terror* (Mark Danner), *The Enemy Combatant Papers: American Justice, the Courts, and the War on Terror* (Karen J. Greenberg, Joshua L. Dratel), *Chain of Command: The Road from 9/11 to Abu Ghraib* (Seymour M. Hersh), *Guantánamo and the Abuse of Presidential Power* (Joseph Margulies), *The Dark Side* (Jane Mayer), *A Question of Torture: CIA Interrogation, from the*

Cold War to the War on Terror (Alfred McCoy), and *Torture Team: Rumsfeld's Memo and the Betrayal of American Values* (Philippe Sands). Human rights groups such as Amnesty International, the Center for Constitutional Rights, Physicians for Human Rights, and Human Rights Watch, and international groups such as the United Nations and the European Union have produced well-documented reports. Most important, a Freedom of Information Act lawsuit filed by the ACLU and other groups secured the release of tens of thousands of pages of documents.

Since the publication of the 2006 edition of *Oath Betrayed*, the administration has been forced to declassify additional documents that give insight into the medical operations in the war on terror prisons. These include:

- The Defense Department Office of Inspector General Review of DoD-Directed Investigations of Detainee Abuse.[27] This report reviews the history of the policies contributing to prisoner abuse and the major investigations of the abuse. It details how the SERE training migrated through psychologists to become part of the interrogation techniques (part 1I, pages 22ff in the review).

- A portion of Admiral Albert Church's investigation of the prisons was discussed in the first edition of this book. In 2008, a few more of the hundreds of pages in this document were declassified.[40] This material discusses medical clearance for interrogation, potentially abusive rectal or genital examinations, interrogator access to medical records, and psychologists' roles in supporting interrogations rather than the mental health of prisoners. It discusses how health care personnel may have misrepresented or failed to report injuries, including lethal injuries.

- Documents obtained by the Senate Armed Services Committee hearing of 2008.[20] The principal organizers (including Major Leso, chair of the BSCT) of coercive interrogation at Guantánamo met on October 2, 2002. They discussed coercive interrogation, the necessity of medical and psychological cooperation, the opposition of law enforcement agencies, and the importance of preventing Red Cross observers from seeing these prisoners, possibly by transferring them to CIA control (pages 14–18 of the online documents). A SERE training visit to the interrogators in December 2002 is described in detail (pages 48–52).

- The interrogation log of Mohammed al-Qahtani. This is a portion of the log of a brutal Guantánamo interrogation that was supervised by a psychologist with the acquiescence of physicians and medics. The document is important because it details how thoroughly medical and psychological experts were integrated into the abuse of prisoners. Appendix 1 of this book includes a discussion guide of this important material.

- Guantánamo Camp Delta Standard Operating Procedures.[41] This indexed and text-searchable 237-page policy describes the rules for concealing prisoners from the International Committee of the Red Cross, limiting exercise to twenty minutes twice per week, and all medical procedures including sick call; management of hunger strikers, death, and suicide; medical records procedures; and the rationing of toilet paper.

- The Department of Justice Office of Inspector General's report on the FBI.[42] This is a detailed review of the FBI's dissent from coercive interrogation in the war on terror prisons, which was briefly outlined in *Oath Betrayed*. Some FBI e-mails on this matter are posted in the ACLU and *Oath Betrayed* web archives.

- In June 2006, the Defense Department issued a new policy responding to concerns about clinical complicity with prisoner abuse.[14] (This replaces the policy discussed on pages 64n144 and 158n61 of this book.) It applies only to prisoners held by the Defense Department and not to those held by the CIA although it is government policy to transfer prisoners to CIA control for special interrogations and to conceal them from the International Red Cross.

Finally, there are documents not from the Defense Department that are essential reading. The Intelligence Science Board of the National Defense Intelligence University report *Educing Information Interrogation: Science and Art* contains four hundred pages and is the current authoritative review of what is known about the science of interrogation. Chapter 2 of the report discusses coercive interrogation's lack of efficacy.[43] Rejali's *Torture and Democracy* is an encyclopedic examination of the history of torture.[23]

AUDIENCES

This book is written for general readers. The inmates of the prisons at Guantánamo Bay, Iraq, and Afghanistan are "prisoners." They are not "detainees," "persons under control" (militarily abbreviated and pronounced PUCs), or "illegal combatants," terms that the government coined in order to try to claim exemption from international norms of civilized conduct.[44-46] Military jargon is explained in brackets, for example, HUMINT [human intelligence]. General readers may ignore superscripted notes, all of which simply give sources rather than elaborate on arguments.

This second edition will be more useful for scholarly readers. Most important, there is now an online archive of all the documents cited in this book. This archive includes tens of thousands of pages of investigations, policies, medical records, and communications from the Defense Department, the White House, and the FBI.[47] The text of this book uses actual names when possible. There are no pseudonyms. Where government censors redacted personal names from documents, I refer to people by job function or rank. The index, which was left out of the first edition because of the rush to publication, is now included. A bibliographic note describes the challenge of citing the unpublished and partly censored government documents.

Scholars may be interested in other online archives of primary source documents on the topic of this book. Table 1 describes major online archives on this matter. Many of these sites offer regular updates. Online archives and listservs are an increasingly powerful human rights tool.[48] They are hampered, however, by inadequate organization and indexing. Such archives can post only what has been declassified or leaked. The CIA rendition and ghost prisoner program remains hidden from sight. The government is destroying interrogation logs in Afghanistan and Iraq and at Guantánamo Bay.

There are two entirely new appendixes. One is a case discussion study guide. The second reviews the policy debate within the American Psychological Association.

TABLE I.1 WEB ARCHIVES ON HUMAN RIGHTS ABUSES IN WAR ON TERROR PRISONS

Name	Description	URL
American Civil Liberties Union	This civil rights group disseminates news of human rights abuses and files legal actions to promote accountability for such abuses. It maintains the largest archive of government documents. The archive is partly indexed and searchable.	http://www.aclu.org/safefree/torture/torturefoia.html
Center for Constitutional Rights	This legal advocacy group tracks court decisions and files legal actions in the United States and Europe to promote accountability for human rights abuses.	http://ccrjustice.org/
Detainee Interrogations, Physicians, & Psychologists	This personally maintained archive contains 300+ citations on psychologist or physician involvement in prisoner interrogation.	http://kspope.com/interrogation/index.php
Human Rights Library: United States Military Medicine in War on Terror Prisons	This personally maintained indexed archive compiles government documents pertaining to clinicians and human rights abuses in war on terror prisons.	http://www1.umn.edu/humanrts/OathBetrayed/index.html
Human Rights First	This human rights group disseminates news of human rights abuses, publishes reports, and engages in activist-focused activities.	http://www.humanrightsfirst.org/
Human Rights Watch	This human rights group disseminates news of human rights abuses, publishes reports, and engages in activist-focused activities.	http://www.hrw.org/
Physicians for Human Rights	This human rights group has a medical focus. It publishes news and reports, and engages in activist-focused activities.	http://physiciansforhumanrights.org/

Name	Description	URL
Psyche, Science, and Society	This blog covers news primarily pertaining to the controversy about the American Psychological Association.	http://psychoanalysts opposewar.org/blog/
Psychologists for Social Responsibility	This human rights group has a psychology focus. It publishes news and reports, and engages in activist-focused activities.	http://www.psysr.org/

PERSONAL REFLECTIONS

I am a practicing physician who teaches internal medicine and medical ethics. My professional life has focused on relieving suffering for persons with chronic diseases, American veterans, and refugees. I have treated Holocaust survivors. As a consultant to the American Refugee Committee, I have worked in countries recovering from war or housing the tortured, bereft refugees of war. I am on the board of the Center for Victims of Torture in Minneapolis. I have lectured or written on torture and human rights in Turkey, the former Soviet Union, South Africa, Cuba, and the United States. These experiences have forged my conviction of the necessity of protecting prisoners from neglect, degradation, and torture. During the past four years of writing and lecturing, I have met many people who struggle on tiny budgets, sometimes at great personal risk, to prevent torture or to treat its survivors. My admiration is unbounded for this small community that holds a candle so we may sense how large the enveloping night of torture is.

Answering the question that engendered this book transformed me. For the first six months, after a day of reading through an endless pile of descriptions of arbitrary brutality, I would dream of being in Abu Ghraib. I would wake up sweating, with my heart pounding. Later, sadness came; I would sometimes stop writing out of a sense of futility. I learned from others in my new field that I was experiencing the secondary trauma that sometimes afflicts those who work in this field.[49] They wisely prescribed family, friends, gardening, and jazz.

By 2006, when *Oath Betrayed* was going to press, I felt anger. I have worked with our soldiers abroad and at a Veterans Administration medical center. Our soldiers are decent people with an honorable history. In this instance, elected officials, secretaries, undersecretaries, and lawyers, along with some military commanders and soldiers, stained institutions and traditions that had been entrusted to their stewardship for safekeeping. As a guest of veterans groups, I have spoken about command responsibility for the abuses at Abu Ghraib and Guantánamo. Our frontline soldiers were betrayed and broken by being tasked with criminal duties. They have been deceived by the Defense Department and Veteran's Administration, institutions that have inadequately responded to the physical and mental consequences of this war. Counterfeit patriotism and bad national security policy deceptively sent our soldiers to war, exposed them to needless risk on the battlefield, and failed to meet their needs when they returned home. This book is dedicated in grief to those who served.

My feelings today are more complex than sadness and anger. I increasingly see the global implications of the human right abuses of the U.S. "war on terror." The U.S. government played a key role in crafting the international laws and standards of decent treatment of prisoners that it has now forsaken. It has forfeited the moral authority to speak for those standards on behalf of prisoners and endangered friends of civil society around the world. Its arguments on behalf of its own policies join with those made by the governments of Zimbabwe and Sudan, which claim that torture is protected by sovereignty and justified by national emergency. As their partners in reasoning and practice, the United States finds its appeals on behalf of human rights answered by jeers from the tyrants of Myanmar. The United States has not fallen alone, but our descent makes it much harder for global civil society to rise.

For this reason, I am increasingly drawn to the need for accountability. My work has made me an ardent proponent of prosecuting war crimes even as it has dispelled most of my hopes for lessening the brutality of battlefields. I am not a pacifist, a fact that may disappoint critics who would pigeonhole and dismiss me and friends who would recruit this work to the cause of pacifism. By prosecuting war crimes and holding those who commit human rights abuses accountable for their actions, we preserve a piece of our humanity during the course of a war and take a small step toward preventing the next one.

***

Many people made this book possible. The Center for Bioethics at the University of Minnesota accommodates my scholarship. Sandra Dijkstra, my agent, prodded me to complete the first edition in a timely manner. Niels Hooper of the University of California Press pushed me to go further with this edition. My wife, Joline, endures and supports my obsessions. With each page, I was mindful that my adoptive son is a refugee from torture-scarred Cambodia. With each word, I knew that my daughters, Esmé and Erica, will live in a world shaped by how we heal and prevent torture's wounds to civil society.

S.H.M.
Minneapolis, Minnesota
August 2008

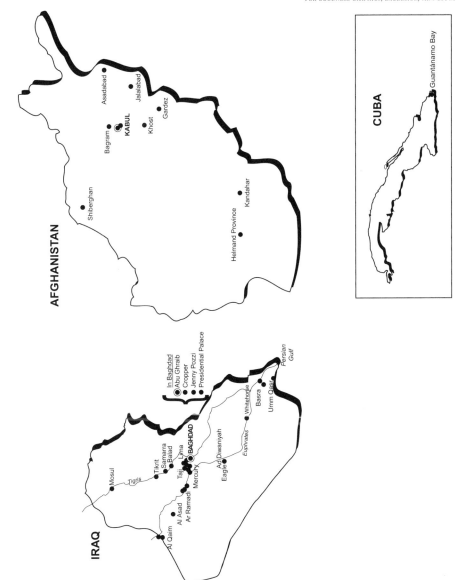

FOR GOODNESS GRAPHICS, EXCELSIOR, MINNESOTA

AFGHANISTAN

Asadabad
Jalalabad
Gardez
Bagram
KABUL
Khost
Shiberghan
Kandahar
Helmand Province

CUBA

Guantánamo Bay

IRAQ

In Baghdad
Abu Ghraib
Cropper
Jenny Pozzi
Presidential Palace

Persian
Gulf

Whitehorse
Basra
Umm Qasr

Mosul
Tigris
Tikrit
Samarra
Balad
Taji Lima
Mercury
BAGHDAD
Ad Diwaniyah
Eagle
Euphrates
Al Asad
Ar Ramadi
Al Qaim

Prisons mentioned in this book.

PART I

"WE ARE SELLING OUR SOULS FOR DROSS"

We receive intelligence obtained under torture from Uzbek intelligence services via the U.S. . . . Tortured dupes are forced to sign up to confessions showing what the Uzbek government wants the U.S. and UK to believe. . . . We are selling our souls for dross.

THE HONORABLE CRAIG MURRAY,
British ambassador to Uzbekistan,
ambassadorial e-mail (July 2004)

CHAPTER 1

TORTURE

IN NOVEMBER 2003, AN IRAQI GUARD SMUGGLED A CHINESE PISTOL into Abu Ghraib and gave it to a prisoner, Ameen Sa'eed Al-Sheikh. An informant promptly told MPs, who locked down the cellblock and began a cell-to-cell search. When they got to his cell, Al-Sheikh went for the pistol hidden in his bedding. Gunfire was exchanged. Sergeant William Cathcart was hit, but not injured, by a ricochet. The soldiers wrestled Al-Sheikh to the floor and sent him to the hospital with a dislocated shoulder and shotgun wounds to his legs.[1] When Al-Sheikh returned to the cellblock after several days in the hospital, Specialist MP Charles Graner beat his wounded leg with a baton while demanding that the prisoner renounce Islam. He then suspended Al-Sheikh by his injured shoulder even though the prisoner's wounded legs could not bear weight to protect the shoulder from further injury.[2,3] Staff Sergeant–Medic Layton Reuben and another medic saw the beating while providing health care in the cellblock.[4,5] On three occasions, Medic Layton found Al-Sheikh handcuffed with his arms over his head, putting stress on his injured shoulder and leg. Each time, he says that he told Graner to remove the handcuffs. Layton considered that to be the extent of his responsibility: he stated, "I feel I did the right thing when I told Graner to get the detainee uncuffed from the bed." Under oath, Medic Layton said that he examined Al-Sheikh in his cell with two officers, a Captain Williams and a physician named Ackerson who held the rank of lieutenant colonel, to confirm that Al-Sheikh had a dislocated shoulder from having his arms handcuffed over his head in his cell. Investigators do not record looking at, or for, the medical record of this examination. There is no evidence that any of these persons reported or tried to stop the abuse, either.[6,7] Months later, an Abu Ghraib investigation recommended that Medic Layton be disciplined for failing to stop or report the ongoing abuse.[8] The released file says nothing about any scrutiny of Dr. Ackerson.

On a cold night, another medic, Sergeant Theresa Adams, saw Al-Sheikh naked and without a mattress or a blanket. The prisoner was bleeding from a drain that should have been connected to a bag to prevent an infection. Sergeant Adams took Al-Sheikh to see the physician on call, who held the rank of colonel. The physician agreed that the hospital had erred in leaving the catheter open but refused to remove the catheter or to transfer Al-Sheikh to the adjoining hospital. When Sergeant Adams asked him whether he had ever heard of the Geneva Convention, the physician answered, "Fine, Sergeant, you do what you have to do; I am going back to bed."[9,10] Later, the physician told investigators that he remembered Al-Sheikh's dislocated shoulder but not the catheter incident, although he agreed that such a catheter should have been removed. That physician also claimed that during four months at Abu Ghraib at the peak of the abusive incidents, he never observed or heard of any abuse, although he did recall the Red Cross complaining about the treatment of the prisoners.[11]

"Torture" comes from the Latin word for "twist," an origin that conveys both a common technique of bending a victim's body or the contortion of a person in agony. The torsion and stretching applied by the medieval "strappado," a ladderlike device that stretched extremities and joints into abnormal and extreme directions, or the shackled "stress positions" widely used in the prisons of the war on terror epitomize the ancient sense of the word. Torture acquired its present meaning of pain inflicted by government officials in France about eight hundred years ago, when the church or governments applied "the torture" to extract confessions or testimony. The English adopted the French noun in about 1550. In 1591, William Shakespeare is credited with first using "torture" as a verb, in *Henry VI*: "Alas, master, I am not able to stand alone: You go about to torture me in vain. [Enter a Beadle with whips]."[12] However, the many appearances of the verb in the years immediately after the play suggest that the Bard simply recorded an existing colloquial use, rather than originating one.

Definitions of torture bear close reading. The UN Convention Against Torture and Other Cruel, Inhuman or Degrading Treatment or Punishment defines torture as

> any act by which severe pain or suffering, whether physical or mental, is intentionally inflicted on a person for such purposes as obtaining from him or a third person information or a confession, punishing him for an act he or a third person has committed or is suspected of having committed, or intimidating or coercing him or a third person, or for any reason based on discrimination of any kind, when such pain or suffering is inflicted by, or at the instigation of, or with the consent or acquiescence of a public official or other person acting in an official capacity.

Similarly, the World Medical Association's "Guidelines for Medical Doctors Concerning Torture and Other Cruel, Inhuman or Degrading Treatment or Punishment in Relation to Detention and Imprisonment" defines torture as

> the deliberate, systematic or wanton infliction of physical or mental suffering by one or more persons acting alone or on the orders of any authority, to force another person to yield information, to make a confession, or for any other reason.

Both of the preceding documents and the Geneva Conventions define torture as a government practice rather than as suffering that is inflicted by a criminal sadist. By defining torture in relation to the reasons that nations use it (for example, to secure information), they emphasize that torture is not justified by any purpose or rationale. Torture is a crime against humanity, but its occurrence is not confined to war: many of the 130 governments that practice torture do so while they are at peace.

Although it is customary to think of torture as a set of techniques, torture is better understood as a social institution. Torturing societies create laws, policies, and regulations to authorize the practices. They establish, empower, and protect specialized practitioners and places. With fear, incentives, and propaganda, they secure the assent or acquiescence of the press, the judiciary, the professions, and the citizenry. This view of torture as an institution means that moral blame may not be simply laid on the individual soldiers or police who employ horrific techniques. Those officials are agents, acting on behalf of national leaders, public policies, and a social and political consensus. Condemning, convicting, or sacrificing low-ranking soldiers as rogues or bad apples neither eradicates nor expiates the crime. Moral responsibility in a torturing society is broadly shared. Reforms and prevention must look up the chain of command and out into the society at large.

THE CASE FOR TORTURE

Governments rationalize torture in various ways. Stalin, Saddam Hussein, and the generals of Argentina's Dirty War used terror to suppress dissent and maintain political control. Hitler used anti-Semitism and the eugenic ideology of "race hygiene" to mobilize a political base and justify genocidal policies. Nigeria amputates the hands of thieves to punish (and putatively deter) crime. Submerging women in water to see whether they floated (guilty of witchcraft) or sank (innocent) is perhaps the most notorious use of torture to answer a question independent of a victim's testimony. The present war on terror rationalizes torture and harsh treatment to facilitate interrogation. In his novel *Waiting for the Barbarians*, the South African writer J. M. Coetzee has a magistrate define faith in interrogational torture this way: "Pain is truth."[13]

There are two general types of coercive interrogation.[14] *Pain interrogation* posits that a person will tell the truth in order to escape pain. Here, a physician may be asked for advice to prevent a prisoner from dying or to ensure that the prisoner remains conscious during questioning. Or a physician might advise on how to decrease the risk of evidential scars or physical disability (the long-term psychiatric consequences of torture, such as post-traumatic stress syndromes, are rarely taken into account). Toward a similar goal of concealing torture, a physician might ensure that medical records or death certificates do not note evidence of trauma. *Psychiatric stress interrogation* endeavors to cause a prisoner to regress and become psychologically dependent on the interrogator. Such captives supposedly become submissive to the interrogator and thereby less resistant to questioning, or less inclined to be deceptive. Here, behavioral scientists, psychiatrists, or psychologists devise plans to psychologically "break" a prisoner without impairing his or her ability to speak the truth. For example, the dose of a barbiturate "truth serum" must be sufficient to relax a prisoner but not so large as to cause an exhausted prisoner to fall asleep or a malnourished prisoner to stop breathing. Alternatively, sensory deprivation must not make a prisoner so psychotic or disoriented that she cannot respond to questions. The techniques encompassed by these two incompletely distinguishable approaches vary according to the torturer's technology and imagination. All are psychologically stressful. Some deprive a prisoner of basic needs. Some cause pain and injury. Most have been used in prisons in the war on terror.

In the "Ethical Issues" section of his investigation of the Abu Ghraib abuses, the former secretary of defense James Schlesinger wrote, "For the U.S., most cases for permitting harsh treatment of detainees on moral grounds begin with some variant of the 'ticking time bomb' scenario. The ingredients of such scenarios usually include an impending loss of life, a suspect who knows how to prevent it—and in most versions is responsible for it—and a third party who has no humane alternative to obtain the information in order to save lives." Mr. Schlesinger continues,

> An excellent example [of a ticking time bomb scenario] is the case of a 4th Infantry Division battalion commander who permitted his men to beat a detainee whom he had good reason to believe had information about future attacks against his unit. When the beating failed to produce the desired results, the commander fired his weapon near the detainee's head. The technique was successful and the lives of U.S. servicemen were likely saved. . . . He was punished in moderation and allowed to retire.[15]

Schlesinger's anecdote is incomplete and misleading—disingenuously so in light of the records of an Army investigation of this incident, completed six months before Schlesinger wrote his report. Those records include an investigative report supported by eight concurring statements

TABLE 1.1 TORTURE PRACTICES[16, 17]

PAIN	DEPRIVATION	PSYCHOLOGICAL
BEATING*	FOOD*	FORCING VICTIM TO ABASE SELF*
Fist*	WATER*	Urinating on self*
Truncheon*	ACCESS TO TOILET*	Masturbating*
Whip	SHELTER FROM HEAT OR COLD*	Renouncing religion*
Kick*	MEDICAL CARE*	Falsely confessing or accusing*
Slamming (against wall, etc.)*	SLEEP*	Applying urine, feces of others*
	SENSORY DEPRIVATION*	
ELECTRICAL SHOCKS		VERBAL ABUSE*
External electrodes*		Threats to the prisoner*
Internal electrodes		Threats against the prisoner's family*
Parilla (strapping a person to electrified metal bedsprings)		Insults*
		Denigration of the prisoner's religion*
STRETCHING OR SUSPENSION* (may tear ligaments or muscles or cause asphyxia)		
		MOCK EXECUTIONS*
ASPHYXIATION*		SEXUAL DEGRADATION*
Water immersion*		Nudity*
Obstructing airway*		Fondling*
Chest compression*		
Suspension*		FORCING A VICTIM TO WATCH ABUSE OR TORTURE OF A LOVED ONE*
BURNING		
Chemical		PERCEPTUAL MONOPOLIZATION*
Thermal*		Loud noise*
LIGATURES		Immobilization*
(e.g., limbs, penis)*		Bright lights/ blindfolding*
RAPE*		Confinement in small space*
PAINFUL MEDICAL PROCEDURES SUCH AS ADMINISTRATION OF DRUGS, ENEMAS, ETC.*		

PAIN	DEPRIVATION	PSYCHOLOGICAL
MUTILATION		DISORIENTING DRUGS SUCH
Dog bites*		AS TRANQUILIZERS OR
Tattoos		HALLUCINOGENS*
Piercing		STEALING INFANTS/
Skinning		CHILDREN
Amputation		

* Practices reliably documented at U.S. detention centers in Iraq, at Guantánamo Bay, or in Afghanistan.

by participating soldiers, among them a sworn statement by Lieutenant Colonel Allen West, clearly describing what happened.[18,19]

Lieutenant Colonel West was never trained to interrogate. He had never even witnessed an interrogation. In August 2003, an Iraqi informant said that Mr. Yehiya Hamoodi, a Shiite police officer working with West's unit, was plotting to ambush West and some of his soldiers. At that time, many Iraqis were giving false tips to the U.S. Army to curry favor or to use the Army to settle their personal gripes. As a military intelligence training slide show used in Iraq at that time put it,

> Personal vendettas against different ethnic groups have caused an influx of bogus reporting from interrogators. . . . Recommendation: Tactical patience is critical when taking action to detain host nation personnel during Stability and Support Operation. It is more of an Art than a Science, and usually learned after the unit makes mistakes.[20]

West promptly sent his soldiers to arrest Mr. Hamoodi. They beat and shackled him and loaded him into their vehicle. When they arrived at the base in Taji, Iraq, they threw him off the Humvee. A medic cleared Mr. Hamoodi for questioning even though his ribs had been hurt by the beating.[21,22]

Soldiers took Hamoodi to an interrogation room. Colonel West told the interrogators that they had one hour to obtain information or he would come down and do it himself. Hamoodi was kicked and beaten by four soldiers for forty minutes. During the latter part of this interrogation, Colonel West sat facing the prisoner with a cocked pistol on his lap that he would occasionally point at Mr. Hamoodi. Colonel West tells how he became increasingly angry and threatened Mr. Hamoodi's life. In a sworn statement, a soldier reported that West told the prisoner, "I have come here for one of two reasons: one, to get the information I need or two, to kill you." A soldier displayed a knife and the translator told Mr. Hamoodi that his toes or fingernails would be cut off if he did not tell the truth. An appalled soldier left the room after reminding West of the Geneva Conventions, an appeal that West rejected. Finally, Colonel West had his soldiers blindfold Hamoodi and escort him outside, where six soldiers surrounded him with guns as the interrogation continued for another fifteen minutes. A translator told Hamoodi, "If you don't talk, they will kill you." West counted down from 10 and shot into the air. Two soldiers forced Hamoodi's head into a barrel. West did another countdown and, angling his gun close to the prisoner's head, fired into the barrel.

Hamoodi became hysterical and "admitted there would be attacks and called out names." A physician's assistant then examined him and found bruises but no serious injuries or bleeding.[23–25] Colonel West's violation of Army interrogation regulations was investigated and charges were filed against him. West then asked to retire.[26,27] Ultimately, he was removed from command, fined $5,000, and allowed to retire with benefits.[28,29] Ninety-five congressional representatives wrote a letter on his behalf. He is fêted with dinners in the United States.[30]

Mr. Schlesinger did not report that no plot was found and that the men whom Hamoodi named were released without being charged.[31] Hamoodi later told investigators that there was no plot and that he gave untrue information.[32]

Mr. Schlesinger also omitted a troubling epilogue to his story. Three months before the Hamoodi incident and in the same area, Master Sergeant Lisa Girman and several soldiers beat and kicked several prisoners at Camp Bucca. At least one detainee was pinned to the ground while soldiers spread his legs and kicked him in the groin.[33,34] Battalion and brigade commanders as well as Army lawyers strongly recommended that the soldiers be court-martialed. A rationale for excusing Colonel West and punishing the Camp Bucca soldiers was that West acted to obtain information for the purpose of "force protection" whereas Girman and her colleagues were simply abusive.[35,36] However, the Army chose not to prosecute some participants in the Girman matter, and it nonjudicially discharged three soldiers. Why did the Camp Bucca abusers get off with such light sanctions? A company commander told Brigadier General Janis Karpinski, who at that time was in charge of Abu Ghraib, "Ma'am, everybody knows that the reason it didn't go to court martial was because they were protecting that Lieutenant Colonel" (of whom Schlesinger wrote so approvingly).[37] Soldiers from that same unit were not retrained in the rules for treating prisoners. Their unit was transferred to Abu Ghraib.[38,39]

Five months later, soldiers from that unit were involved in the photographed abuses at Abu Ghraib.[40] As Major Michael Sheridan, the commanding officer of the 800th Military Police Brigade at Abu Ghraib, later put it, if those soldiers had "been court martialed . . . you never would have had another incident after that. [It] . . . was a crime and [the involved soldiers] should have been made to pay for it."[41]

Mr. Schlesinger cut and polished the story of Colonel West to create a "ticking time bomb" fable for torture. But in his "excellent example," torture alienated an Iraqi who had been working with the U.S. forces, and it arguably contributed to tolerance of torture in the unit that became responsible for the photographed abuses at Abu Ghraib.

A similar disregard for the facts shapes accounts of the interrogation of the terrorist Abdul Hakim Murad, who reportedly disclosed a plot to blow up eleven trans-Pacific airliners after being successfully tortured.[42] Investigators actually learned of the plot from his computer files, not by torturing him.[43]

Fictional dramas of the *Mission: Impossible* or 24 genre present a seductive case for "ticking time bomb" scenarios, with syncopated music, countdown digital clocks, and flashing cutaways to innocent victims, their loved ones, the tense rescuers, and a prettified harsh interrogation. Real interrogations rarely, if ever, contain the combination of elements that must come together for the "ticking time bomb" scenario to be realized. Interrogators rarely know whether a given prisoner has foreknowledge of a specific and imminent crime. Even if a prisoner knows about a future crime, that information is rarely of immediate utility to interrogators. Analysts must fit the prisoner's knowledge into a larger puzzle, a process that usually takes a considerable amount of time. The "ticking time bomb" scenario resembles an anecdote in Dostoevsky's novel *The Brothers Karamazov*. Ivan poses this question to his brother, a young priest, Alyosha.

> Imagine that you are creating a fabric of human destiny with the object of making men happy in the end, giving them peace and rest at last, but that it was essential and inevitable to torture to death only one tiny creature — that baby beating its breast with its fist, for instance — and to found that edifice on its unavenged tears, would you consent to be the architect on those conditions?[44]

Ivan's fanciful question is cynically crafted to compel Alyosha to accept the utilitarian conclusion that a baby could be tortured for the sake of social good. The "ticking time bomb" scenario is similarly constructed to justify torture, not to illuminate the moral issues of legalizing torture. Charles Krauthammer, who is a political commentator, a psychiatrist, and a member of President George W. Bush's Council on Bioethics, writes, "If you have the slightest belief that hanging this man by his thumbs will get you the information to save a million people, [not] only is it permissible to hang this miscreant by his thumbs, it is a moral duty. . . . And even if the example I gave were entirely hypothetical, the conclusion [that] in this case even torture is permissible . . . establishes the principle. . . . [To] paraphrase George Bernard Shaw, all that's left to haggle about is the price."[45] Dr. Krauthammer smoothly glides from his justification for torture to prevent a nuclear attack, to using torture to identify a suicide bomber who plans to go into a coffee shop, to torturing an accomplice who may have information about the whereabouts of a single uniformed soldier. His "slightest belief" standard is the political rhetoric that has often been used to rationalize the murder, torture, and disappearance of millions of innocent or ignorant people.

An honest inquiry into the wisdom of legalizing torture would build from realistic moral questions for policymakers. Is it justifiable to torture one person to save a thousand innocent lives? Ten? Two? Is it ethical to torture any person allegedly "affiliated" with a criminal group, on the assumption that he or she possesses knowledge that can be used to avert a crime? Should interrogational torture be limited to situations where strong evidence points to an imminent attack, or may it be applied to an inchoate or long-range fear of possible attack? Is it moral to use interrogational torture knowing that most of those questioned will be innocent or ignorant? If so, how should society balance the harms to those people against the good that allegedly comes from torture? Should society compensate or provide therapy to the innocent victims of legal torture? Is it moral to torture a culpable person who is unlikely to give useful information despite being tortured? Is it smart to torture when torture procures false information that swamps the limited resources available for intelligence analysis? Is it wise to employ torture when torture is likely to make our enemies more numerous and harden them against us?

Advocates for legal torture have grappled with some of these questions.[46] They argue that, since the "ticking time bomb" scenario is plausible, however rare, it would be naïve, idealistic, and irresponsible to ban torture's use.[47,48] Some propose procedural safeguards (such as torture warrants), by which courts would weigh the gravity or probability of the crime that interrogational torture would endeavor to prevent.[49] Some suggest that torture should remain illegal but that courts should allow an after-the-fact "necessity" defense, somewhat like allowing a person to claim the necessity of homicide in self-defense. History does not justify confidence in such measures. Twentieth-century torture has always spread far beyond "ticking time bomb" scenarios to result in the abuse of many innocent or ignorant persons. Societies that torture light the fuse on a real time bomb. It is naïve, idealistic, and irresponsible to claim otherwise.

THE CASE AGAINST INTERROGATIONAL TORTURE

1. Torture Harms Intelligence Collection and Analysis

The U.S. Central Intelligence Agency's Clandestine Services Department sponsored eleven years of research on interrogation in Project

MK-ULTRA during the Cold War.[50-52] When MK-ULTRA ended in 1964, the CIA continued the research under Project MK-SEARCH for another decade. The primary aims of this research were (1) to develop ways to train American personnel to resist coercive interrogation and (2) to determine whether the Soviets, Koreans, or Chinese could brainwash prisoners along the lines of Richard Condon's 1959 potboiler *The Manchurian Candidate*, in which a POW is programmed to assassinate a U.S. presidential candidate. CIA-funded researchers studied Korean, Chinese, and Soviet interrogation. They conducted about two hundred studies examining the use of hypnosis, stress, electric shock, coma, sensory deprivation, sedatives, hallucinogens (including LSD), drugs that induced symptoms to mimic diseases or disabilities, or sensory deprivation to improve interrogation. The agency destroyed the individual project reports, but Richard Helms, who oversaw the research, testified to Congress that it had been unproductive. A declassified CIA "Counterintelligence Interrogation Manual" from 1963 refers to MK-ULTRA's findings:

> The threat of death has often been found to be worse than useless. . . . No report of scientific investigation on the effect of debility upon the interrogatee's power of resistance has been discovered. For centuries, interrogators have employed various methods of inducing physical weakness: prolonged constraint; prolonged exertion, extremes of heat, cold or moisture; and deprivation or drastic reduction of food or sleep. Apparently, the assumption is that lowering the source's physical resistance will lower his psychological capacity for opposition. . . . Prolonged exertion, loss of sleep, etc., themselves become patterns to which the subject adjusts through apathy. . . . Interrogatees who are withholding but who feel qualms of guilt and a secret desire to yield are likely to become intractable if made to endure pain.[53]

The CIA's "Human Resource Exploitation Manual" of 1983 came to the same conclusion: "Use of force is a poor technique. . . . However, the use of force is not to be confused with psychological ploys, verbal trickery, or other nonviolent and non-coercive ruses." The "Army Interrogation Field Manual" of 1987 reiterated these same conclusions.[54]

The governments of Nazi Germany, China, North Vietnam, Great Britain, and Israel also found pain to be an unreliable interrogation technique. As prisoners disintegrate, harden, or dissociate under pain, they tend to give inaccurate, useless, or misleading information. Although American POWs subjected to psychiatric stress by Korean, Chinese, or Soviet captors seemed to be more willing to make anti-American statements while in captivity than those who were tortured with pain, there is no evidence that psychological torture improved the ability to get the truth from a prisoner.[55]

Advisers to Secretary of Defense Donald Rumsfeld informed him of the research showing the inefficacy of harsh interrogation.[56] The secretary then authorized the same harsh techniques that had been discredited by the research and experience of the United States.

From 2003 to 2004, as poorly trained and inexperienced Army interrogators were brutally applying Rumsfeld's "counterresistance" techniques, experienced interrogators were complaining about the abuses and citing the conclusion of the CIA's 1983 "Human Resource Exploitation Manual" ("Use of force . . . can induce the source to say what he thinks the interrogator wants to hear") as they complained about the Army interrogators. An FBI interrogation instructor, Joe Navarro, said that threats "taint information gained from sessions. . . . The only thing that torture guarantees is pain, it never guarantees the truth."[57] Roger Bokroas, a retired military interrogator, tried to stop harsh treatment at Abu Ghraib and later testified, "Whenever you use harsh treatments you are more likely to get false information just to stop the treatment."[58,59] In their Guantánamo interrogation debriefing memos, many FBI agents expressed skepticism of the truth of statements that prisoners made under duress.[60–65] One FBI interrogator wrote, "He was taken to the 'dark place.' At the 'dark place,' a hood was placed over his head and he was yelled at and beaten. [Name redacted] stated that because of this treatment at the hands of his captor, he provided the interrogators with whatever information that they wanted to hear."[66] Craig Murray, then the British ambassador to Uzbekistan, sent a diplomatic cable protesting harsh interrogations conducted for the United States:

> We receive intelligence obtained under torture from Uzbek intelligence services via the U.S. We should stop. It is bad information anyway. Tortured dupes are forced to sign up to confessions showing what the Uzbek government wants the U.S. and UK to believe. . . . I repeat that this material is useless—we are selling our souls for dross.[67]

False information elicited by pain floods the limited analytic capacity of intelligence agencies. As the CIA's KUBARK interrogation manual put it, "pain is quite likely to produce false confessions, concocted as a means of escaping from distress. Time-consuming delay results, while investigation is conducted and the admissions are proven untrue." In this way, harsh interrogation can make it more, not less, difficult for analysts to find "ticking time bombs." Torture seeks and tends to elicit information that exaggerates the size and nature of the threat. Such false information can lead to misguided government policies. The CIA illegally flew the Al Qaeda operative Ibn-al-Shaykh al-Libi to Cairo. Under torture, he became an authoritative source for what Secretary of State Colin Powell, President Bush, and Vice President Dick Cheney claimed as "credible" evidence that Iraq was training Al Qaeda members in the use of explosives, poisons, and gases. Mr. al-Libi has since recanted his inaccurate confessions.[68]

Torture alienates persons who might otherwise be recruited as informants. As the CIA's 1983 "Human Resource Exploitation Manual" put it, "Use of force . . . may damage subsequent collection efforts." Many FBI reports of interrogations with prisoners in the war on terror tell of prisoners who refused to cooperate with interrogators because of harsh, abusive, or degrading treatment meted out to fellow prisoners or themselves.[69–79] Some prisoners even experience torture as validating their sense of importance, the rightness of their cause, or, conversely, the evil of their torturer. For example, some Palestinian prisoners tortured by Israelis experienced torture as a rite of passage that bonded them to their cause, confirmed the evil of Israel, and proved their trustworthiness to comrades.[80–82]

Abusive interrogation fosters an "arms race" between interrogators and prisoners. As targeted groups learn the techniques that will be used against their members, they prepare their colleagues for what to expect. They take measures to limit the amount of damaging information that any individual can disclose. As interrogators change in reaction to the strategic moves of prisoners, the targeted organizations adapt again.

Effective interrogation seeks to build rapport, articulate common interests, exploit a subject's jealousy of comrades, or offer, in exchange for information, something that the prisoner sees as being in his or her interest. Torture destroys the possibility of this kind of interview. The abuse hardens the prisoner's political commitment and perception of the interrogating authority. An interrogator who abuses a prisoner forfeits the emotional self-control that is necessary for effective interrogational interviewing.[83]

2. Torture Is Strategically Counterproductive

Coercive interrogation is especially ineffective in asymmetrical warfare between a regular army and guerrillas living among an indigenous population of sympathizers who are familiar with the insurgents' factions and social organizations. Terrorist profiling cannot identify the key persons in such communities.[84] Hundreds of citizens have mere bits of knowledge. Dragnets for coercive interrogation are expensive and ineffective. Military Intelligence personnel estimate that from 70 percent to 90 percent of the tens of thousands of Iraqi prisoners were either innocent or ignorant.[85–88] Proponents of interrogational torture cite the occasional tactical success of French soldiers who used torture to learn of terrorist attacks during Algeria's war for independence from France.[89] However, those same abuses alienated the Algerian population and fueled the resistance; France lost the war.

A similar pattern is unfolding in Iraq. The revelations of abuses in U.S. prisons were followed by a dramatic decline in international respect for the United States and a sharp increase in anti-American sentiment, especially in the international Muslim community.[90,91] U.S. government polls found that Iraqi support for U.S. forces fell from 63 percent to 9 percent upon the release of the Abu Ghraib photographs.[92] It seems probable that interrogational torture in Iraq boosted insurgency recruitment and resulted in far more attacks than it could have prevented.

3. TORTURE HARMS THE SOCIETY THAT EMPLOYS IT

Torturing societies harm their courts, their militias, and the officials who torture on their behalf. The Defense Department and FBI knew that evidence obtained by coercive interrogation could not be used in prosecuting either the person who gave the information or those implicated by that interrogation.[93] The inadmissibility of that evidence is part of why the FBI dissociated itself from harsh interrogations.[94]

The 1983 CIA "Human Resource Exploitation Manual" asserts: "Torture lowers the moral caliber of the organization that uses it and corrupts those that rely on it as the quick and easy way out." In 2003, Defense Secretary Rumsfeld's Working Group on Detainee Interrogations warned him, "Participation by U.S. military personnel in interrogations which use techniques that are more aggressive than those appropriate for POWs would constitute a significant departure from traditional U.S. military norms and could have an adverse impact on the cultural self-image of U.S. military forces."[95]

Torture psychologically traumatizes the soldiers who perform it. Soldiers who passively witness atrocities, as well as those who commit them, suffer more severe post-traumatic stress disorder than those who kill during combat.[96,97] Abu Ghraib medics were providing Prozac and starting Alcoholics Anonymous groups for soldiers in the abusive units.[98] It is reasonable to expect painful scars in the soldiers who participated in prisoner abuse. Those wounds will burden their lives, their families, our neighbors, our society, and the Veterans Administration for years to come.

TORTURE AND AMERICAN CULTURE

In *Regarding the Pain of Others*, Susan Sontag wrote that powerful images of violence, pain, or suffering are "like a quotation, a maxim, or a

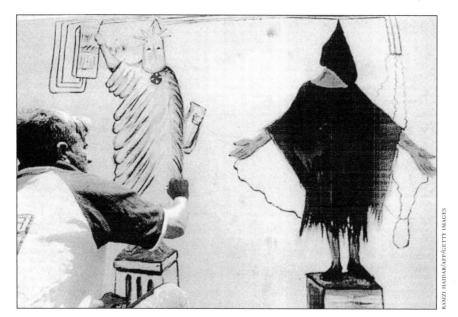

FIGURE 1.1. *Iraqi artist Sala Edine Sallat at work.*

proverb."[99] She noted that the terse captions supplied with such photographs seem to expect the viewer to supply the interpretation that a visceral reaction demands. "Prisoners and Guards at Abu Ghraib" was a typical news caption of a photograph of a pyramid of bruised, naked men with their heads in sandbags (it illustrates Chapter 6, "Silence"). Other captions are possible. For this book on medical complicity with torture, the caption might read, "What the nurse saw while working at Abu Ghraib."

Americans are fascinated with images of torture even though we carefully keep its frightful reality at a distance. Our favorite form of voyeurism is fictional torture. Astonishing quantities of American cinema, television shows, video games, and books are built with the elements of torture. A torturer has a twisted sense of entitlement. A victim is isolated and controlled. The techniques are sadistic, violent, terror-inducing, and often sexually stimulating to torturer and voyeur alike. The urbane Hannibal Lecter walks with the outlandish Freddy Krueger, the buffoonish Goldfinger, and the executive sociopath Patrick Bateman of *American Psycho*. This phenomenon is not recent. Exquisite Renaissance paintings depict

Christian martyrs posed in orgiastic death throes. Who can forget the terrified monologue that is Poe's "The Pit and the Pendulum"? Children's television is a kindergarten of torture-themed cartoons which, it might be charitably said, recapitulate the plots of trapped and endangered children in the European fairy tales collected by the brothers Grimm. Madame Tussaud's Wax Museum, amusement park horror rides, and Halloween houses all offer torture as 3-D entertainment.

Fiction is one way to keep torture at a distance; the censorship of images of real torture is another. Movies may show graphic degradation because they are fiction. However, the same corporations that produce those movies primly sanitize torture for their news shows. The Abu Ghraib photographs show brutally beaten bodies, even the faces of corpses, with tastefully pixilated buttocks and genitals. The U.S. government would not release photographs showing the degradation of Iraqi women and children; news organizations that obtained leaked versions declined to show them.[100] Only elected officials were allowed to see the Abu Ghraib videos.

Given our fascination with torture, it is surprising that no image of torture has acquired the stature of other iconic images of human violence, degradation, and despair. Until Abu Ghraib, no photograph of torture is as instantly recognized as that of the naked, napalm-seared Vietnamese girl, Phan Thi Kim Phuc, running toward the camera—toward us, who had sent that napalm to her village. That image came to symbolize the cruelty of that war, of war itself. It is not that photographers have been barred from places of torture. The Nazis and the Khmer Rouge kept large photographic archives. Photographs of South American torture victims have been used to humiliate or blackmail victims, extort money from families, or intimidate others. The guards of Abu Ghraib are not the only soldiers to stage "photo opportunities" for personal gratification.[101] Even an American medic paused during his work to be photographed pointing an M-16 rifle at a wounded prisoner's head while making an obscene gesture: he intended to "keep [the photo] as a souvenir of what I did here in Iraq."[102] The absence of iconic images of real torture is another sign of how carefully we maintain a distance between real torture and our daily life. The Abu Ghraib photographs annihilated that gap with a thunderclap of horror that echoed throughout the citizenry and government.

Americans looked at the photographs to see American soldiers looking back at them through the camera lens, not as victims, not as rescuers, but as smiling tormentors.

Real torture challenges the moral passivity of armchair voyeurs of fictional torture. It does not provide the comforting certainty that the half-hour cartoon, the one-hour police drama, or the two-hour movie will end by uncovering a reason for torture and bring the perpetrator to justice (usually after some innocent secondary characters are disposed of along the way). Real torture forces the viewer to make a political judgment rather than an artistic evaluation such as "That was a gripping movie."

Although every civilized person at some level condemns torture, each person's reaction to real torture that penetrates the careful distancing of fictional and foreign torture will vary according to historical perspective and experience. It is ironic that when 60 *Minutes* televised soldiers' *amateur* photographs from Abu Ghraib it forced elected officials, citizens, and news media to confront the truth of *authoritative* written reports that they had ignored for two years. Even then, some Americans dismissed the photographs. Conservative commentator Rush Limbaugh told his "ditto-heads" that the events were like "anything you'd see Madonna or Britney Spears do on stage."[103] Some Americans responded with hostility. People spat on and assaulted a California gallery owner who exhibited Guy Colwell's paintings depicting scenes from Abu Ghraib prison. Other artists, such as Andres Serrano and Fernando Botero, have incorporated images from Abu Ghraib into their work.[104,105] The artist Jenny Holzer projected excerpts from the government's torture memos on the exterior walls of New York University's Bobst Library, less than two miles from the site of the fallen World Trade Center towers. An immense, insubstantial pall of dissembling words reflects off an institution epitomizing respect for language and civil society.[106]

In the Arab world, the images from Abu Ghraib have also provoked powerful responses. In Jordan, Muhammad Shawaqfa's popular play, *A New Middle East*, is staged with prison bars between the audience and the actors. The dialogue contrasts sardonically amused soldiers with anguished victims as the action moves from tableau to tableau, reenacting the Abu Ghraib photographs. A lavishly made Turkish movie, *Valley of the* Wolves — *Iraq*, shows American soldiers crashing a wedding and killing the groom along with dozens of guests. A child is shot in front of his mother. The surviving guests are taken to Abu Ghraib, where their organs are taken for rich people in New York, London, and Tel Aviv.[107] In Iraq, the photographs have inspired street and gallery art such as that shown on page 19. The Muslim cleric Sheik Mohammed Bashir said of the photographs,

> It was discovered that freedom in this land . . . is the freedom of the occupying soldiers to do what they like. . . . No one can ask them what they are doing, because they are protected by their freedom. . . . No one can punish them, within our country or their country. They express the freedom of rape, the freedom of nudity and the freedom of humiliation.[108]

These diverse reactions to images and text from Abu Ghraib reveal a common revulsion to the abuses even as they show how viewers' cultural and psychological perspective profoundly shapes their conclusions about the meaning and significance of the images.

The American consciousness has been traumatized by these photographs. Like all peoples, we minimize or deny our atrocities: lynching, Jim Crow, the genocide of Native Americans, or the violence that is allowed to occur within our prisons. A century of support for torturing societies in Europe (for example, Great Britain in Northern Ireland), Africa (for example, apartheid-era South Africa), South and Central America (for example, Argentina, Chile, El Salvador, Guatemala), the Middle East (for example, Israel, Egypt, Turkey), and Southeast Asia (for example, Vietnam, Indonesia) should temper any American claim to the moral high ground with regard to torture. Even so, the fact that it was allies and proxies who committed such acts allowed the people of the United States to deny or minimize their national complicity. Comforting rationalizations, such as the notion of "realpolitik," essentially said, "Those (brutal, uncivilized) people in (corrupt, unstable, or potentially Communist) countries (always or must) torture; is it not so?" Such distancing left Americans unprepared for how easily the plague could infect the homeland.

The Abu Ghraib photographs showed that the United States had become infected. Americans recoiled with new denials. Torture by American soldiers must be a different kind of torture: "torture lite." It must be an isolated event, the work of a "few bad apples" or a local command breakdown. It surely was a response to unusual provocation; the world changed with 9/11. The prisoners are terrorists by definition; they deserved what they got.

None of these denials is true.

The United States is a torturing society.

CHAPTER 2

MEDICINE AND TORTURE

HEALERS AND TORTURERS HAVE HAD A PROFESSIONAL PARTNERSHIP for at least five hundred years. Sixty years ago, the world's reaction to Nazi physicians' horrific abuse of death camp prisoners finally drove a wedge between torture and the ethics of medicine. Sadly, that postwar medical ethic has more voice than power. Torturing societies routinely employ doctors and nurses to work in their prisons. They use fear, political incentives, and propaganda to secure the acquiescence of civilian medical societies and to marginalize medical opponents to torture. Twenty to fifty percent of torture survivors report that they saw physicians serving as active accomplices during the abuse.[1,2] That statistic does not include prisoners who never see the physician who falsifies medical records or death certificates so as to conceal torture. It does not count those who are victimized by techniques that doctors and psychologists devised for torturers to use.

Notwithstanding this grim assessment, history seems to be edging away from torture. For centuries, torture was a discretionary prerogative of powerful individuals. In the European Middle Ages, it was legalized and reserved for duly authorized officials. In the eighteenth century, it was legally abolished. When it reemerged in the twentieth century, it no longer had legitimacy; although widespread, it was stigmatized and illicit, and it had to remain clandestine. Governments that engage in torture risk being sanctioned; their senior officials may be tried for crimes against humanity. Even low-ranking torturers are pursued and may face criminal or civil prosecution, with no international sanctuary from a statute of limitations. The historical movement, especially the movement away from medical complicity with legal Renaissance torture and toward medical partnership with illicit twentieth-century torture, forms the background for understanding and evaluating the actions of American military health professionals in the present war on terror. The active and passive complicity of American military medical personnel with the abuse and neglect of prisoners in Iraq, in Afghanistan, and at Guantánamo Bay renewed a partnership of healers and abusers that dishonored American military medicine.

LICIT TORTURE

Torture has been practiced by diverse societies throughout recorded history. Its oldest use was to punish enemies and criminals. Ancient Greece used torture to interrogate slaves; Rome extended that practice to freemen.[3] The Medieval church invented the strappado, a frame that suspended a person so that a torturer could apply five increasingly severe degrees of stretching and twisting to his limbs and back. The strappado engendered the term "interrogation by the third degree," in that torsion to the fourth degree was lethal.[4] The fifth degree is not described, but records suggest it referred to dismemberment.

During the Renaissance, physicians were assigned legal roles in interrogational torture.[5,6] The German Constitutio Criminalis Carolina, of 1532, required a physician to certify that a person was not incapable of giving testimony by virtue of being blind, mute, or insane and that he or she could survive a planned regimen of torture. By confirming pregnancies, midwives afforded a temporary exemption from torture for women. Such medical and midwifery certificates were used throughout Europe until torture became illegal during the eighteenth century. As long as torture was legal or ecclesiastically licit, "torture physicians" were not stigmatized, secretive, or coerced.[7]

Torture became illegal in Europe when the public concluded that it was inherently barbaric, subject to abuse, and an unreliable way to secure evidence. Ironically, the Habsburg empire's 1769 publication of the Nemesis Theresiana penal code, which was written to reform the arbitrary use of torture and other punishments, fueled revulsion at the techniques of torture and hastened legal abolition.

Enlightenment intellectuals across Europe argued that torture was irrational and violated the inherent dignity of persons. Although Voltaire is better known, the most influential compilation of arguments against torture appeared in *Of Crimes and Punishments* (1764) by the Italian prison reformer Cesare Beccaria.

> The impression of pain, then, may increase to such a degree, that, occupying the mind entirely, it will compel the sufferer to use the shortest method of freeing himself from torment . . . and he will accuse himself of crimes of which he is innocent: so that the very means employed to distinguish the innocent from the guilty will most effectually destroy all difference between them. . . . The examination of the accused is intended to find out the truth; but if this be discovered with so much difficulty in the air, gesture, and countenance of a man at ease, how can it appear in a countenance distorted by the convulsions of torture? Every violent action destroys those small alterations in the features which sometimes disclose the sentiments of the heart. . . .
>
> [A] necessary consequence of the use of torture is, that the case of the innocent is worse than that of the guilty. . . . [The first either] confesses the crime which he has not committed, and is condemned, or he is acquitted, and has suffered a punishment he did not deserve. On the contrary, the person who is really guilty has the most favourable side of the question; for, if he supports the torture with firmness and resolution, he is acquitted, and has gained, having exchanged a greater punishment for a less.[8]

The seventeenth-century French writer Jean de La Bruyère described the rack as "a marvelous invention and an unfailing method of ruining an innocent weakly man and saving one who is robust and guilty."[9]

The English jurist William Blackstone scorned torture as an "inhuman species of mercy" in his famed *Commentaries on the Laws of England*: "It seems astonishing [to be] . . . rating a man's virtue by the hardiness of his constitution, and his guilt by the sensibility of his nerves."[10] Physicians also criticized the reliability of statements obtained under torture but apparently did not claim that medical complicity with torture violated their profession's ethics. Public acceptance of the moral and utilitarian arguments against torture led to its legal abolition.

As legal torture was ending in Europe, two physicians took a step that foreshadowed a new role that medical professionals would assume in facilitating twentieth-century torture. They applied their medical stature and insight to promote and design a penal technique. In 1789, the physician and legislator Dr. Joseph-Ignace Guillotin gave a famous speech before the French revolutionary legislature advocating an antitorture law and proposing other penal reforms, among them that

> in all cases where the law imposes the death penalty on an accused person, the punishment shall be the same, whatever the nature of the offence of which he is guilty; the criminal shall be decapitated; this will be done solely by means of a simple mechanism.

Previously, prominent persons were more likely to be swiftly beheaded (although a clumsy executioner or dull blade sometimes botched the job) while ordinary people were more likely to be executed by painful methods, such as being broken on the wheel, burned alive, or quartered. Dr. Guillotin argued for equitably minimizing the pain of execution, but he did not invent the decapitation machine. The Halifax gibbet, the Scottish maiden, and other diverse instruments had been used throughout Europe for at least four centuries. After Guillotin's law was enacted, a surgeon, Dr. Antoine Louis, designed France's penal decapitator. He proposed that the ax should be a heavy, diagonal-cut blade of a specified weight. He detailed that the blade was to be mounted in a frame so that it would fall smoothly and accurately and slice cleanly. The device was tested on corpses that were obtained from a prison hospital. The French device was briefly called a *louisette* or *louison* in honor of its inventor but was soon called the more euphonious *guillotine* in honor of its proponent. Contrary to legend, Dr. Guillotin was not beheaded; he died of an infected pimple.[11] His descendants changed their name to dissociate themselves from the stigma.

ILLICIT TORTURE

Legal abolition did not end torture. It drove the practice underground during the nineteenth century, until it exploded into sight as a global crime against humanity in the twentieth century. In torture's modern incarnation, physicians took on the same duties as their ancestral Renaissance colleagues. They certified that prisoners could withstand torture. An El Salvadoran prisoner tells how two persons "introduced themselves as doctors. They examined me, and checked me all over. One of them said to me that 'you must put up with it' . . . then they both left," whereupon his interrogators began to administer electric shocks.[12] Physicians monitored persons being tortured and advised interrogators on adjusting the severity of treatment so that the prisoner could be punished or interrogated without dying, losing consciousness, or becoming psychotic. A Chilean prisoner recounts how a physician periodically ordered that his torture be paused and drugs administered whenever his blood pressure became too high. Iraqi physicians guided the torture of prisoners at Abu Ghraib under Saddam Hussein.[13] The presence of a physician during torture compounds the victim's suffering by emphasizing that even the humanity of medicine is turned against the prisoner.

Twentieth-century physicians built on the precedent set by Drs. Guillotin and Louis of applying medical knowledge to the punishment of prisoners. The transitional act was to employ medical knowledge to refine capital punishment. American physicians and medical societies promoted electrocution as an alternative to hanging and supervised research to design electric chairs.[14] Nazi physicians devised a variety of ways to euthanize chronically ill Germans before the Holocaust.[15] More recently, American physicians created protocols for execution by lethal injection and assisted in the punishment.[16] Extending the nontherapeutic use of medical knowledge, military physicians and behavioral scientists studied how to use psychoactive, hallucinogenic, and caustic drugs and sensory deprivation to cause pain, anxiety, disorientation, or regression.[17] Nazi physicians adjusted food rations so that prisoners could work as they were economically starved to death.

Given the illicit nature of modern torture, physicians took on two roles that were unnecessary during legal torture. They helped government officials develop physical and psychological techniques that would not leave incriminating wounds. To the same end of protecting torturers from accountability, physicians failed to record signs of torture on medical reports and death certificates.[18] In 1979, interrogators sent a Chilean teacher to the Penitentiary Hospital in respiratory distress with "multiple contusions on the cranium, thorax and extremities." The dying man was transferred to an intensive care unit with a death certificate that had been written and signed in advance. It stated, "The undersigned physician has professionally examined Federico Renato Alvarez Santibañez . . . and found him in good health and showing no wounds of any kind."[19] Dr. Hussain Majid, Saddam Hussein's chief physician at Abu Ghraib, ensured that death certificates failed to record the executions of political prisoners.[20]

Physician-torturers do not have a unique psychological profile.[21] The psychiatrist Robert Jay Lifton proposes that Nazi physicians resolved the moral contradiction of being a healer and a torturer by "doubling"—that is, by developing a genocidal professional self and a normal world self that enabled them to be loving parents and good, even religious, citizens.[22] Doubling may characterize some torturing physicians, but it seems unlikely to characterize most of them. Nazi physicians, such as Josef Mengele, joined the party early and were committed to its eugenic pseudoscience that ennobled physicians as "public health" practitioners of "race hygiene."[23] Mengele unabashedly combined his political and medical passions by supervising mass selections for execution and sadistic "experiments" at Auschwitz. Dr. Andrei Snezhnevsky, the director of the Soviet Union's Institute of Psychiatry, aggressively defended the practice of diagnosing dissidents with the counterfeit disease "sluggish schizophrenia" and committing such "mentally ill" persons to asylum-prisons where they were abused with drugs and brain surgery.[24] Sometimes, membership in a medical profession seems entirely incidental to the role of torturer. Radovan Karadžić, a Serb psychiatrist turned politician, managed concentration camps where torture, rape, starvation, and summary executions were routine.[25] Coercion or threats are rarely necessary to secure the services of physician-torturers; most are simply thoughtless careerists. Dr. Claudia Malzfeldt, a victim and scholar of East German torture, has said, of East German physicians who betrayed their patients in this way, "It is clear that they were not monsters who worked there. Most doctors were probably just doing their job as far as they could. . . . They didn't have to do it. To say no, you didn't have to be a hero."[26] Most physicians who abet torture simply rationalize their work. A Uruguayan psychiatrist who collaborated with torture put it this way: "I was confined to my function. I ignored some aspects and there were some aspects I didn't want to know about. . . . It wasn't my purpose. I am a doctor."[27] Likewise, a Chilean physician who served during Pinochet's reign of terror dismissed the moral contradiction of torture and medicine thus: "What do you expect? We are at war."[28]

Any history of medicine and torture must note sadistic experiments on prisoners. Sometimes, this included research to develop new interrogational techniques. Sometimes, it served other state research interests. It always exploited the simple expendability of prisoners. In the first century, King Mithridates of Asia Minor poisoned prisoners in order to test antidotes to protect himself from assassination.[29] Celsus, a first-century Roman, wrote that the Egyptian anatomists Herophilius and Erasistratus, who lived three centuries earlier, had

> laid open men whilst alive—criminals received out of prison from the kings—and whilst these were still breathing, observed parts which beforehand nature had concealed, their position, color, shape, size, arrangement, hardness, softness, smoothness, relation, processes and depressions of each and whether any part is inserted into another or received into another.[30]

Celsus' censure expresses his first-century moral judgment of abusive research on prisoners, even though it is probably a historically inaccurate slander. Nazi physicians conducted horrific experiments on concentration camp prisoners. Prisoners were frozen to test cold-water survival gear; subjected to sudden decompression to test aircraft depressurization suits; shot or infected with germs to simulate battlefield trauma; and exposed to chemical weapons. Some prisoners, even children, were killed and dissected to validate racist theories or to develop anatomical atlases or museum exhibits. Nazi physicians performed experiments using mescaline for interrogation; the CIA conducted similar research with LSD. During World War II, Japanese physicians performed vivisection on prisoners whom they had exposed to biological warfare agents.[31]

In sum, physicians and psychologists collaborate with torturers in six ways. Some examine prisoners to certify them as capable of withstanding harsh interrogation. Some monitor and treat persons during interrogation so that health-endangering treatment may proceed. Some conceal evidence of abuse, either by designing nonscarifying techniques or by ensuring that medical documents or death certificates do not record injuries. Some conduct abusive research. Some oversee the systematic neglect of prisoners' needs for health care, sanitation, food, and shelter. Many keep silent as their imprisoned patients are abused. This investigation examines whether and how the actions of U.S. medical personnel who worked in the foreign military prisons of the war on terror fit into this historical context.

OPPOSING TORTURE

The trials of Nazi leaders at Nuremberg for war crimes and crimes against humanity revealed the immense scale of that regime's atrocities. Those trials engendered international laws to outlaw genocide and to protect prisoners from torture, abuse, and neglect. Through the newly created United Nations, the international community reiterated the Enlightenment conclusion that torture was inherently barbaric and could not be justified by appealing to investigative necessity, war, national sovereignty, or revenge. The 1948 UN Universal Declaration of Human Rights captures the spirit of this time and its moral, rather than utilitarian, rejection of torture:

> Whereas the peoples of the United Nations have . . . reaffirmed their faith in fundamental human rights, in the dignity and worth of the human person . . .
>
> Now, therefore, the General Assembly proclaims this Universal Declaration of Human Rights as a common standard of achievement for all peoples and all nations. . . .

Article 5: No one shall be subjected to torture or to cruel, inhuman or degrading treatment or punishment.

The Universal Declaration of Human Rights became the cornerstone of international and national covenants, laws, and regulations banning torture and cruel, inhuman, or degrading treatment or punishment.[32] The global community endorsed the similarly unequivocal language of the Geneva Conventions a year later:

> Persons taking no active part in the hostilities, including members of armed forces who have laid down their arms and those placed hors de combat by sickness, wounds, detention, or any other cause, shall in all circumstances be treated humanely. . . .
>
> To this end, the following acts are and shall remain prohibited at any time and in any place whatsoever with respect to the above-mentioned persons: (a) Violence to life and person, in particular murder of all kinds, mutilation, cruel treatment and torture; . . . (c) Outrages upon personal dignity, in particular humiliating and degrading treatment. . . .*

The 1975 Final Act of the Conference on Security and Co-operation in Europe, also known as the Helsinki Accords, reaffirmed the Universal Declaration of Human Rights. The International Covenant on Civil and Political Rights, passed by the United Nations in 1966, is as unambiguous as English can be.

> *Considering* that, in accordance with the principles proclaimed in the Charter of the United Nations, recognition of the inherent dignity and of the equal and inalienable rights of all members of the human family is the foundation of freedom, justice and peace in the world,
>
> *Recognizing* that these rights derive from the inherent dignity of the human person,
>
> *Recognizing* that, in accordance with the Universal Declaration of Human Rights, the ideal of free human beings enjoying civil and

*Citations to other documents, with Web addresses, appear in the bibliography.

political freedom and freedom from fear and want can only be achieved if conditions are created whereby everyone may enjoy his civil and political rights, as well as his economic, social and cultural rights. . . .

Agree upon the following articles . . .

Article 7: No one shall be subjected to torture or to cruel, inhuman or degrading treatment or punishment.

The Achilles' heel of all of these documents is the lack of a means to hold nations accountable for any breach of their commitments. The eighteenth-century experience with abolishing torture suggested that nations would abandon torture only if they saw it as *both* barbaric and ineffective. The post–World War II sentiment against torture is unstudiously oblivious to the kind of research discussed in the preceding chapter and so it stood on moral argument alone.

World revulsion at medical collaboration with torture was ignited by revelations of the actions of Nazi physicians at death camps. In 1946 and 1947, twenty-three physicians were indicted, tried, and mostly convicted at Nuremberg for war crimes and crimes against humanity pertaining to their complicity in mass murder and in sadistic experiments on prisoners.[33] Ironically, the United States shielded equally barbaric Japanese physicians from prosecution because "the value to the U.S. of Japanese biological warfare data is of such importance to national security as to far outweigh the value according from war crimes prosecution."[34] Even so, the trials of Nazi doctors ensured that physician complicity with the abuse and neglect of prisoners would become a special problem for medical ethics.

After the war, the international community and private medical societies soon began to develop ethical standards for physicians who were responsible for the well-being of prisoners. In 1948, a year after the Nuremburg trials, but before ratification of the Geneva Conventions, the World Medical Association, a congress of national medical associations, adopted its Declaration of Geneva. In this professional oath, physicians promise, "I will not use my medical knowledge contrary to the laws of humanity." In addition to banning torture and inhuman treatment, the 1949 Geneva Conventions and the 1955 UN Standard Minimum Rules for the Treatment of Prisoners set minimal standards for medical oversight respecting the shelter, food, sanitation, and medical care provided for prisoners. In 1956, the World Medical Association issued a more explicit document, Regulations in Time of Armed Conflict.

> The primary task of the medical profession is to preserve health and save life. Hence it is deemed unethical for physicians to: give advice or perform prophylactic, diagnostic, or therapeutic procedures that are not justifiable in the patient's interest [or to] weaken the physical or mental strength of a human being without therapeutic justification.

The World Medical Association's 1956 regulations were clearer than its 1948 Declaration of Geneva but still only obliquely referred to the partnership of health professionals with torture.

In the 1970s, there were renewed efforts to explicitly assert that complicity with torture violated medical ethics. Amnesty International's 1973 Conference for the Abolition of Torture made a stab at it: "Medical and associated personnel shall refuse to allow their professional or research skills to be exploited in any way for the purpose of torture, interrogation, or punishments nor shall they participate in the training of others for such purpose." In 1975, the World Medical Association passed the landmark Declaration of Tokyo (formally, the Guidelines for Medical Doctors Concerning Torture and Other Cruel, Inhuman or Degrading Treatment or Punishment in Relation to Detention and Imprisonment):

> The doctor's fundamental role is to alleviate the distress of his or her fellow men, and no motive whether personal, collective or political shall prevail against this higher purpose.
>
> The doctor shall not countenance, condone or participate in the practice of torture or other forms of cruel, inhuman or degrading procedures, whatever the offence of which the victim of such procedure is suspected, accused or guilty, and whatever the victim's belief or motives, and in all situations, including armed conflict and civil strife. The doctor shall not provide any premises, instruments, substances or knowledge to facilitate the practice of torture or other forms of cruel, in-

human or degrading treatment or to diminish the ability of the victim to resist such treatment. The doctor shall not be present during any procedure during which torture or other forms of cruel, inhuman or degrading treatment are used or threatened.

The Declaration of Tokyo annulled the illegitimate partnership between medicine and torture. In 1982, the UN responded to the Declaration of Tokyo with its Principles of Medical Ethics Relevant to the Role of Health Personnel, Particularly Physicians, in the Protection of Prisoners and Detainees against Torture and Other Cruel, Inhuman or Degrading Treatment or Punishment:

> Principle 2: It is a gross contravention of medical ethics, as well as an offence under applicable international instruments, for health personnel, particularly physicians, to engage, actively or passively, in acts which constitute participation in, complicity in, incitement to or attempts to commit torture or other cruel, inhuman or degrading treatment or punishment. . . .
>
> Principle 6: There may be no derogation from the foregoing principles on any ground whatsoever, including public emergency.

Using the Declaration of Tokyo as a model, other medical societies proceeded to pass their own codes condemning medical complicity with torture.[35–41] For example, the International Council of Nurses statement recapitulates the history of these documents in defining nursing ethics.[42]

> The International Council of Nurses (ICN) supports the United Nations Universal Declaration of Human Rights. Furthermore, we declare: The nurse's primary responsibility is to those people who require nursing care. Nurses have the duty to provide the highest possible level of care to victims of cruel, degrading and inhumane treatment. The nurse shall not voluntarily participate in any deliberate infliction of physical or mental suffering. . . . ICN further advocates that national nurses' associations develop mechanisms to ensure nurses have access

to confidential advice and support in caring for prisoners sentenced to death or subjected to torture.

In 1996, the World Psychiatric Association issued its Declaration of Madrid stating that "psychiatrists shall not take part in any process of mental or physical torture, even when authorities attempt to force their involvement in such acts."[43]

U.S. medical associations adopted their own statements against medical participation in torture. The Ethics Manual of the 100,000-member American College of Physicians, for example, is clear: "Physicians must not be a party to and must speak out against torture or other abuses of human rights." The American Medical Association's Council on Ethical and Judicial Affairs passed this standard:

> Torture refers to the deliberate, systematic, or wanton administration of cruel, inhumane, and degrading treatments or punishments during imprisonment or detainment. Physicians must oppose and must not participate in torture for any reason. Participation in torture includes, but is not limited to, providing or withholding any services, substances, or knowledge to facilitate the practice of torture.
>
> Physicians must not be present when torture is used or threatened. Physicians may treat prisoners or detainees if doing so is in their best interest, but physicians should not treat individuals to verify their health so that torture can begin or continue. . . .
>
> Physicians should help provide support for victims of torture and, whenever possible, strive to change situations in which torture is practiced or the potential for torture is great.

In the 1980s, medical opposition to torture was buttressed by research showing that torture had persistent ill effects on survivors. In addition to physical injuries, especially to the shoulders, ears, and lower back, many torture survivors suffer long-lasting psychiatric disabilities. The term "post-traumatic stress disorder" (PTSD) does not convey the full effects of torture on a person's emotional, social, and occupational life.[44-48] Many torture survivors experience nightmares, flashbacks, depression, apathy, anxiety, phobias, and impaired concentration and memory. Torture often creates persistent difficulties establishing trusting or intimate relationships. Survivors may withdraw from social life and they are at increased risk of suicide. The two hundred torture-victim treatment centers around the world also found that medical complicity with torture can engender a profound fear of medical professionals that deters survivors from seeking or trusting those who would help them to heal.

Knowledge from research with torture survivors has been incorporated into newer medical ethics codes, for example, the 1985 statement by the American Psychiatric Association and the American Psychological Association, which states:

> Whereas, psychological knowledge and techniques may be used to design and carry out torture, and . . . whereas, torture victims often suffer from multiple, long-term psychological and physical problems, be it resolved, that the American Psychiatric Association and the American Psychological Association condemn torture wherever it occurs.[49]

As with the international laws against torture, it is one thing to pass a medical ethics code and quite another to enforce it.

The biggest barrier to enforcement is a lack of political will on the part of governments and medical societies. Governments routinely shield their medical accomplices from prosecution. Judicial proceedings arising from crimes of torture focus on soldiers.[50] International war crimes tribunals focus on national and military leaders and rarely pursue clinicians. The sanctioning of torture-abetting clinicians is left to medical societies and licensing boards. Unfortunately, civilian medical organizations in torturing societies too often condemn such complicity in principle while remaining passive in fact with regard to their colleagues who abet torture.

Professional sanctions against medical personnel are rare enough to be noteworthy. The Medical Council of São Paulo, Brazil, revoked Dr. Harry Shibata's medical license for falsifying the death certificate of torture victims while he was the director of the Forensic Medical Institute.[51] Uruguay's National Medical Council suspended five physicians for complicity with torture.[52] The World Medical Association has called on governments to suspend the licenses of physicians accused of torture until the allegation is cleared.[53] The United Kingdom is the only country to have enacted a law to this effect.

Some medical societies oppose their own governments in order to sanction clinicians. In such cases, international human rights organizations, such as Physicians for Human Rights or Amnesty International, often campaign on behalf of medical societies or practitioners who are at risk because of their opposition to torture. General Augusto Pinochet's junta took control of the Chilean Medical Association in 1973. Under an "antiterrorist" statute, the police threatened and imprisoned medical personnel who were suspected of treating or supporting "subversives." Upon reacquiring the ability to elect its own officers, the Chilean Medical Association expelled six physicians for supervising torture. The regime responded by organizing its own medical society to enroll and license the expelled physicians.[54] The Turkish Medical Association has steadfastly resisted torture despite pressure from the government and disappointing behavior by some Turkish physicians.[55,56] Drs. Cumhur Akpinar, Seyfettin Kizilkan, and Zeki Uzun are among the many Turkish physicians and nurses who have been arrested for their work against torture and supported by the medical association. Dr. Uzun was arrested for documenting injuries. His files were seized. He was kept in isolation, deprived of sleep, interrogated, beaten, and kicked on the head and chest. A plastic bag was placed over his head to induce the feeling of suffocation. A bottle was inserted into his rectum and his testicles were squeezed. He has explained his actions this way: "I have been loyal to the Hippocratic Oath . . . and I will continue to perform my profession."[57]

Where medical societies will not act, individual practitioners, sometimes at great personal risk, act alone. Dr. Anatoly Koryagin, a Soviet psychiatrist, was imprisoned for twelve years for publishing a medical journal article, "Patients Against Their Own Will," about the political abuse of psychiatry in the Soviet Union. After being forced into exile, he said, "I can't be silent when people are kept in psychiatric hospitals for their political beliefs. We can't live on our knees like slaves when they do these things."[58,59] In South Africa, security police beat to death Steve Biko, a black civil rights leader and medical student, after arresting him under an antiterrorism law.

Police physicians failed to record or treat his injuries. Dr. Frances Ames, of the University of Cape Town, complained to the National Medical Board. The board, which was embedded in the apartheid regime and culture, tabled the complaint. Eight years later, the South African Supreme Court demanded an investigation that resulted in one physician being reprimanded and another having his license temporarily suspended.[60,61]

In 1976, Paraguay's government viewed Dr. Joel Filartiga's "Clinic of Hope" for poor people as a subversive organization. Police kidnapped Dr. Filartiga's son, Joelito, and beat, whipped, and electrocuted him to death. One of Joelito's torturers immigrated to the United States, where the family successfully sued him for emotional damages.[62]

There are other means to hold physicians accountable for collaborating with torture. In 1996, international human rights advocates stopped a leader of the Rwandan genocide from practicing obstetrics in Belgium.[63] Sometimes vigilantism prevails. A Chilean army major, Dr. Carlos Pérez Castro, was murdered along with his wife soon after the Chilean Medical Association found that he had falsely certified the good health of prisoners who had been tortured to death.

U.S. military medical personnel have a largely honorable tradition of service, skill, and respect for the human rights of prisoners. Most of those who have treated prisoners during the war on terror aspired to provide good care. The following chapters discuss cases in which military health professionals failed to uphold the ethics of their profession; their lapses are similar to the lapses of colleagues in other torturing societies. Enough practitioners complied when they should have resisted, or kept quiet when they should have spoken out, to allow abusive interrogational practices and a neglectful prison environment to operate largely without medical opposition or disclosure. Although few military physicians, nurses, or medics were explicitly familiar with ethics standards bearing on work in military prisons, even an uninformed sense of professional responsibility asked more of them. No U.S. armed forces' medical professional faced risks comparable to those borne by such colleagues as Doctors Filartiga, Koryagin, and Uzun for professional advocacy on behalf of abused and neglected prisoners whose health was their responsibility.

The history of medical complicity with torture shows that it was possible to anticipate and therefore prevent the medical abuse and neglect that are described in this book. The failure to teach that history to medical professionals lies with health professional societies and with civilian and military medical educators. The failure to incorporate the lessons of that history into prison policy lies with senior military officers and officials.

PART II

"TANTAMOUNT TO TORTURE"

In these cases, persons deprived of their liberty under supervision of military intelligence were at high risk of being subjected to a variety of harsh treatments ranging from insults, threats and humiliations to both physical and psychological coercion, which in some cases was tantamount to torture in order to force cooperation with their interrogators.

International Committee of the Red Cross,
February 2004

CHAPTER 3

INTERROGATION

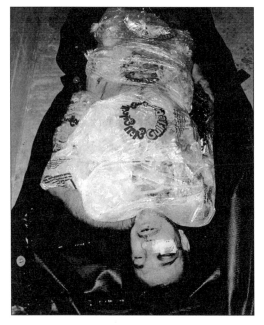

FIGURE 3.1. *The iced body of Monadel al-Jamadi.*

THE INTERROGATION OF MONADEL AL-JAMADI

AT TWO A.M. ON NOVEMBER 4, 2003, SEAL TEAM 7 ARRESTED
Monadel al-Jamadi at his home near Baghdad as a suspect in attacks
against U.S. forces.[1,2] As his family looked on, he fought the soldiers. The
SEALs shackled him and flipped him into the back of their Humvee;
they beat, kicked, and sat on him during the short ride to an Army base.[3]
An hour later, he was taken to a SEALs base, Camp Jenny Pozzi. There,
he was threatened and interrogated in the "romper room" as a medic,

Jerrod Holferty, watched. Al-Jamadi was groaning, "I'm dying; I'm dying." The interrogator responded, "You will be wishing you were dying." Al-Jamadi did not receive medical evaluation or care. He was again thrown into a Humvee and this time taken to Abu Ghraib. Despite beatings, kicks, and a "butt stroke" to his head from a riflestock, Al-Jamadi walked into the prison; his head was enclosed in a sandbag, he was naked below the waist, and he was shaking from the cold, fright, and fatigue. He was having difficulty breathing. He was not admitted to Abu Ghraib as a normal military prisoner. Instead, the CIA imprisoned him as a "ghost" prisoner, meaning that his name was not registered and that, despite his injuries and complaints, he did not receive the customary medical examination given to new prisoners.[4,5] The SEALs turned him over to the CIA at five A.M.[6]

Under CIA supervision, Al-Jamadi's arms were bound together behind his back. A shackle running from a barred shower-room window to his wrists lifted his arms up behind his back during the interrogation.[7] If he fell down, his arms would be wrenched backward and upward in the shoulder sockets. This technique is called Palestinian hanging, because it has reportedly been used by Israelis; however, it has also been used by Turkey and other nations as well.[8] At trial, the CIA said that testimony as to whether a cloth soaked with water was placed over Al-Jamadi's face to induce air hunger was classified. After a short interrogation, Al-Jamadi fell down. A CIA interrogator called guards, telling them, "This guy does not want to cooperate." Guards came and tried to lift the wrist shackles behind Al-Jamadi's back higher. The prisoner's arms were bulging backward out of the shoulder sockets. Blood came from his mouth. Al-Jamadi was dead weight.[9]

The sandbag was now taken off his head. Al-Jamadi's eyes were fixed open; he was dead. An Iraqi physician working with the CIA pronounced the death. That unidentified doctor may have been Hussain Majid, who was medical director of Abu Ghraib under Saddam Hussein, when the prison was used for torturing and executing political opponents. Dr. Majid was working as a senior physician at Abu Ghraib for the U.S. government when Al-Jamadi died.[10] Military intelligence and CIA personnel were upset that Mr. Al-Jamadi had died before giving information.

Captain Donald Reese, commander of the Abu Ghraib guards, came to the shower room to hear Colonel Thomas Pappas, commander of military intelligence, say, "I am not going down for this alone." CIA personnel ordered that the corpse be kept overnight in a shower room.[11,12] Lieutenant Colonel Steven Jordan was sent to get ice. As Sergeant Ivan "Chip" Frederick wrote in an e-mail, "They stressed him out so bad that the man passed away. They put his body in a body bag and packed him in ice for about 24 hours." The reason for binding the body with duct tape and packing it in ice remains unexplained. Sabrina Harman and other members of the military police posed for photographs with the body packed in the melting ice.[13] The next day, a medic inserted an IV in the corpse's arm and guards rolled the body out of the prison on a gurney, as if Al-Jamadi were merely ill. Colonel Pappas says that this ruse was designed so as to "not upset the other detainees." The Army Surgeon General's investigation accepts Colonel Pappas's word that it was not an attempt to conceal the manner or time of death.[14,15] Vice Admiral Albert Church, however, concluded that medical personnel might have been attempting to conceal the homicide.[16] Interrogators at Abu Ghraib were told that Al-Jamadi died of a heart attack.[17,18]

The Armed Forces Institute of Pathology helped conceal the homicide. Five days after the death, institute pathologists conducted an autopsy and concluded that Al-Jamadi had died of "blunt force injuries complicated by compromised respiration."[19] The autopsy and death certificate were not released to the Red Cross to give to the family even though the Navy had taken Al-Jamadi from his home. The homicide became public knowledge after CBS's 60 *Minutes* news program ran photographs of Al-Jamadi's corpse with other Abu Ghraib pictures five months later. Four weeks after the CBS show, the Armed Forces Institute of Pathology finalized and released the six-month-old death certificate. Although Mr. Al-Jamadi had been arrested in front of his wife and children, his body was sent to the Baghdad morgue, where it lay unclaimed for at least six months. If it remained unclaimed, it was destined for an unmarked grave in Najaf's Valley of Peace cemetery.[20]

The commanding officer of the SEALs platoon that beat Al-Jamadi before imprisonment was acquitted of responsibility for the death. Eight soldiers received administrative punishments or reprimands for abusing Al-Jamadi and other prisoners handled by that unit. The senior CIA or Army officials responsible for Al-Jamadi's treatment at Abu Ghraib have not been sanctioned. The medic who inserted the IV in the corpse was apparently not reprimanded.

"THE GLOVES ARE COMING OFF"

In mid-2003, U.S. forces in Iraq faced intensifying resistance. Nearly three hundred American soldiers had died. The Pentagon demanded better intelligence on the organization, strategy, and tactical priorities of the resistance. In mid-August, Captain William Ponce of military intelligence sent a message to an e-mail list for intelligence personnel soliciting their "wish list" of interrogation techniques from field officers. He wrote:

> The gloves are coming off gentlemen regarding these detainees. Colonel Boltz has made it clear that we want these individuals broken. Casualties are mounting and we need to start gathering info to help protect our fellow soldiers from any further attacks. I thank you for your hard work and your dedication.
> MI [military intelligence]
> ALWAYS OUT FRONT.[21,22]

Reactions to Ponce's two A.M. request came swiftly. The first reaction was from an officer who forwarded Ponce's e-mail to others in his unit, "Sounds crazy, but we're just passing this on."[23] An unidentified major recognized the danger of Ponce's attitude and promptly sent this breathtaking rebuttal to the same listserve.

> As for "the gloves need to come off . . ." we need to take a deep breath and remember who we are. Those gloves are . . . based on clearly established standards of international law to which we are signatories and in part the originators. . . . It comes down to standards of right and wrong—something we cannot just put aside when we find it inconvenient. . . . "The casualties are mounting . . ." we have taken casualties in

every war we have ever fought—that is part of the nature of war. . . . *That in no way justifies letting go of our standards* [emphasis in original]. . . . BOTTOM LINE: We are American soldiers, heirs of a long tradition of staying on the high ground. We need to stay there.

[Signature redacted]

Psalm 24:3–5 [Who shall ascend the hill of the LORD? And who shall stand in his holy place? Those who have clean hands and pure hearts, who do not lift up their souls to what is false, and do not swear deceitfully. They will receive blessing from the LORD, and vindication from the God of their salvation.][24]

Other interrogation officers in Tikrit, Iraq, interpreted Ponce's request as a green light to test the limits on interrogation. Ideas came in, including this response from an intelligence official:

Today's enemy . . . understands force, not psychological mind games or incentives. I propose a baseline interrogation technique that at a minimum allows for physical contact resembling that used by SERE ["Survival, Evasion, Resistance and Escape": a program to train American POWs how to resist harsh interrogation] instructors. This allows open handed facial slaps from a distance of no more than about two feet and back handed blows to the mid section from a distance of about 18 inches. . . . I also believe that this should be a minimum baseline. Other techniques would include close confinement quarters, sleep deprivation, white noise and a litany of harsh fear-up approaches . . . [ellipses in original] fear of dogs and snakes appear to work nicely.[25]

The 4th Infantry's final wish list included blows with phone books, low-voltage shock, closed-fist blows, and so on.[26] A month later, General Raymond Odierno, commanding the 4th Mechanized Infantry in Tikrit where Ponce's memo circulated, reminded his troops, "Neither the stresses of combat, nor deep provocation will justify inhumane treatments. Such ill treatment of detainees is a serious crime, punishable under international law and the Uniform Code of Military Justice."[27] Even so, a month after General Odierno's memo, Captain Ponce's e-mail was cited in defense of a soldier charged with beating the soles of a prisoner's feet with a baton.[28]

Secretary of Defense Rumsfeld sent Major General Geoffrey Miller from Guantánamo to Iraq to beef up the military intelligence there. General Miller visited Abu Ghraib, Saddam Hussein's notorious prison, which was being used as a detention center for common criminals and suspected insurgents. He liked its proximity to U.S. facilities in Baghdad. He brushed aside the reservations of Brigadier General Janis Karpinski about converting the understaffed frontline prison under her command into the premier joint intelligence and detention facility in Iraq. She pointed out that she had only 300 MPs to defend the besieged prison and to supervise 7,000 prisoners, whereas Miller's Guantánamo was not subject to attack and had 800 guards for 640 prisoners. Miller told her, "You have to have full control. . . . You have to treat these detainees like dogs. If you treat them any differently and they get the idea that they're making decisions or they're in charge, you've lost control of the situation."[29] Finally, Miller told Karpinski, "I want you to give me Abu Ghraib." She replied, "Sir, Abu Ghraib is not mine to give you." Miller cleared the room, faced Karpinski, and told her, "Look, we can do this my way or we can do this the hard way. . . . [General Ricardo] Sanchez [commander of Coalition ground forces in Iraq] said I could have whatever facility I wanted and I want Abu Ghraib."[30]

Miller's plan was to "GITMOize" Abu Ghraib—that is, to make it resemble the interrogation center that he had managed at Guantánamo Bay, "GITMO." His jargon-laden field report proposed to "rapidly exploit internees for actionable intelligence . . . [and to] improve the velocity and operational effectiveness of counter-terrorism interrogation."[31,32] General Sanchez and Colonel Pappas, commander of the 205th Military Intelligence Brigade in Iraq, implemented the Guantánamo model with a potentially significant, but ultimately inconsequential, variation: although President Bush had decreed that the Geneva Conventions did not apply to prisoners in Afghanistan or Guantánamo, the Geneva Convention Relative to the Protection of Civilian Persons in Time of War was official policy with respect to prisoners in Iraq.[33] Despite this, it is hard to find a discernible difference between the abusive imprisonment and treatment in Convention-bound Iraq and Convention-free Afghanistan and Guantánamo. Prison commanders, soldiers, civilian interrogators, and medical personnel did not know, or were not trained in, their human rights obligations.[34–37] Arab synopses of the Conventions were not posted in cellblocks in Iraq, as required by the Conventions and by Army regulations.[38]

General Sanchez and Colonel Pappas remade Abu Ghraib as an interrogation center. Military personnel and "special agents" without name tags came from Guantánamo and Afghanistan to assist in the project. Wooden interrogation rooms with observation windows were constructed.[39] The doors and windows of Cellblock IA were covered with plywood to prevent common criminals from seeing into the living quarters for prisoners being interrogated. That newly private space was where the infamous Abu Ghraib photographs would be taken. According to most testimony, General Karpinski had been ineffective and out of touch as the senior commander of Abu Ghraib MPs. By late 2003, that made no difference. When Abu Ghraib became an interrogation center, she essentially commanded the building but not its staff. Captain Reese was responsible for the prison guards. Army Intelligence devised interrogation plans, which it and the guards jointly administered. The CIA independently admitted unregistered ghost prisoners. A third of the interrogators were civilians. Janis Karpinski with her one-star brigadier generalship had one job left: ranking scapegoat.

Abu Ghraib became a prison without an exit. Mobile Interrogation Teams, which were supposed to screen people at the point of arrest, simply forwarded the captives to prison. As one military intelligence officer put it, "It seemed that the maneuver units gave very broad instructions to round up any male from 16 to 60 years of age that has a cell phone without another verification that they were a bad guy. . . . In my opinion, less than 10% of the detainees had any real intelligence value."[40] Other Army personnel estimated that 80 percent to 90 percent of arriving Abu Ghraib prisoners either had no intelligence value or were outright innocent.[41–46] By February 2004, Abu Ghraib's population of common criminals, suspected insurgents, and intelligence targets had swelled to 7,500 persons.[47] The Military Intelligence Unit, designed for 300 prisoners, held 900.[48] The overcrowding stressed prisoners and guards alike. As one new group of detainees arrived, General Karpinski complained to Major General Walter Wojdakowski, the second-highest-ranking general in Iraq, "I am not going to cram more tents into the compound. The secret here is getting these people released and we're holding innocent people out there."[49] Wojdakowski replied, "I don't care if we're holding 15,000 innocent civilians! We're winning the war!" Karpinski said, "Not inside the wire, you're not, sir."

General Karpinski describes the Army as afflicted with "releaseophobia."[50] It feared that freed prisoners would attack U.S. troops. In response to another group of arriving, and largely innocent, prisoners, General Sanchez reportedly said, "Why are we detaining these people; we should be killing them."[51]

In late 2003, Colonel Stuart Herrington, who was asked to assess the military intelligence operation in Iraq, assessed the effect of detaining large numbers of Iraqis: "Between the losers and dead end elements from the former regime and foreign fighters, there are enough people in Iraq who already don't like us. . . . Adding to these numbers by conducting sweep operations . . . is counterproductive to the Coalition's efforts to win the cooperation of the Iraqi citizenry. Similarly, the mistreatment of captives as has been reported to me and our team is unacceptable and bound to be known by the population."[52] His assessment was prophetic. In early 2006, the military leadership in Iraq was deeply worried that the overcrowded prison had become "a graduate-level training ground for the insurgency." The new strategy was to try to avoid sweeps that dumped prisoners into Abu Ghraib. As one American officer put it, "We don't want to be putting everybody caught up in a sweep into Jihad University."[53]

MEDICALLY INFORMED INTERROGATION PLANS

The interrogation system was built from the top down. At the top, Secretary of Defense Rumsfeld's interrogation directives prescribed medical complicity in counterresistance interrogation (for further discussion, see Chapter 7, "Grave Breaches"). As his directive moved down the chain of command, it was translated into policies and orders which in turn became routines that were then modified on the fly. The policies and practices migrated from one theater to another.[54] Miller carried the GITMO model to Iraq. Captain Carolyn Wood designed a poster for Abu Ghraib based on her work as military intelligence commander at Bagram prison in Afghanistan. Captain Wood's poster summarized rules for coercive interrogation that ironically (or perhaps sardonically) mentioned that the Geneva Conventions applied; but the Geneva Convention on Prisoners of War states:

> No physical or mental torture, nor any other form of coercion, may be inflicted on prisoners of war to secure from them information of any kind whatever. Prisoners of war who refuse to answer may not be threatened, insulted, or exposed to any unpleasant or disadvantageous treatment of any kind.

Captain Wood's poster stated the substance of Rumsfeld's policy for medical oversight of harsh interrogations: "Dietary Manip (monitored by med)" and "Wounded or medically burdened detainees must be medically cleared by med prior to interrogation."[55] (See Figure 3.2.)

It is possible to discern the operation of the system for medical clearance for interrogations. In late 2004, an Air Force medical team consisting of a physician's assistant, two medics, and a technician under Major Karyn Ayers, a board-certified physician in family medicine, claimed to have examined each Abu Ghraib detainee before and after interrogation.[56] However, in 2005, the Army's Surgeon General found that only 15 percent to 50 percent of prisoners in Iraq, Afghanistan, and Guantánamo Bay were examined before interrogations and that less than 15 percent were examined for injuries after questioning.[57] The use of Air Force personnel for interrogation exams supposedly eliminated a conflict of interest that would have existed if Army personnel had medically cleared prisoners for interrogation, questioned them, and then examined them for ill effects afterward.[58,59] This Army–Air Force arrangement did not, however, remedy the nontherapeutic purpose of the medical examinations. The exams were not for the benefit of the prisoners' health; rather,

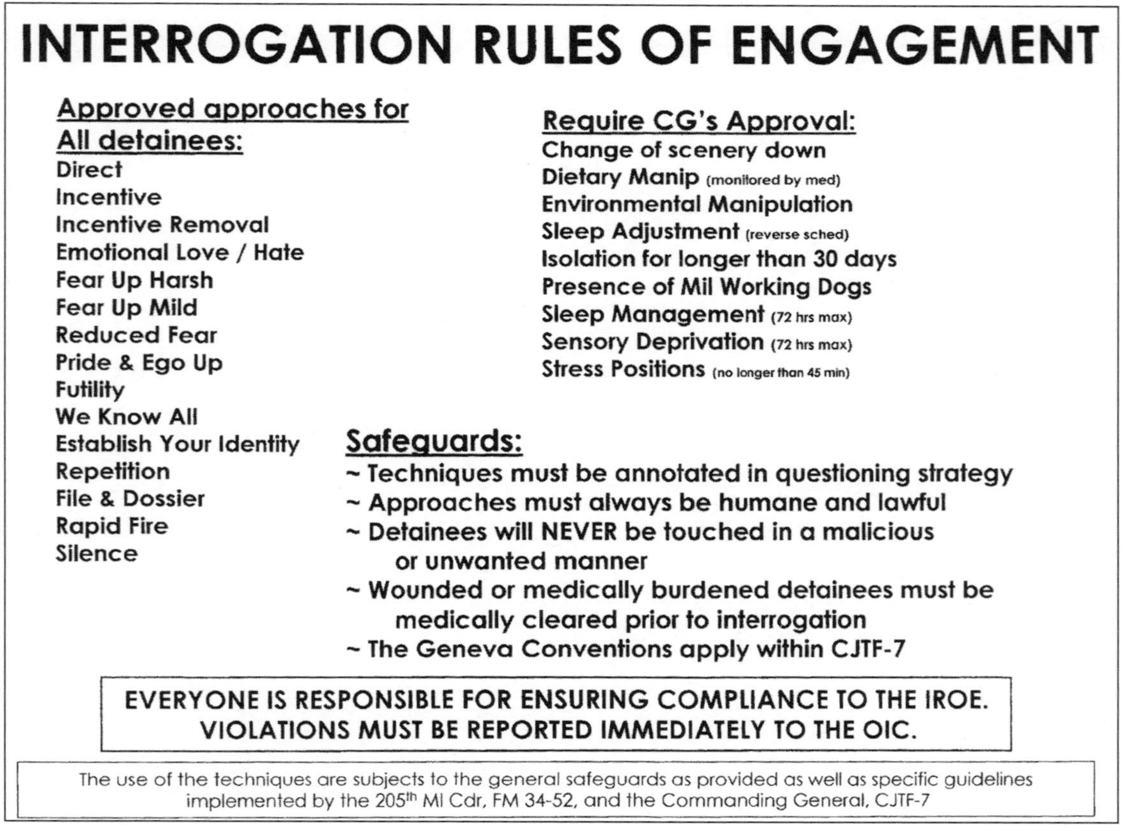

INTERROGATION RULES OF ENGAGEMENT

Approved approaches for
All detainees:
Direct
Incentive
Incentive Removal
Emotional Love / Hate
Fear Up Harsh
Fear Up Mild
Reduced Fear
Pride & Ego Up
Futility
We Know All
Establish Your Identity
Repetition
File & Dossier
Rapid Fire
Silence

Require CG's Approval:
Change of scenery down
Dietary Manip (monitored by med)
Environmental Manipulation
Sleep Adjustment (reverse sched)
Isolation for longer than 30 days
Presence of Mil Working Dogs
Sleep Management (72 hrs max)
Sensory Deprivation (72 hrs max)
Stress Positions (no longer than 45 min)

Safeguards:
~ Techniques must be annotated in questioning strategy
~ Approaches must always be humane and lawful
~ Detainees will NEVER be touched in a malicious
   or unwanted manner
~ Wounded or medically burdened detainees must be
   medically cleared prior to interrogation
~ The Geneva Conventions apply within CJTF-7

**EVERYONE IS RESPONSIBLE FOR ENSURING COMPLIANCE TO THE IROE.
VIOLATIONS MUST BE REPORTED IMMEDIATELY TO THE OIC.**

The use of the techniques are subjects to the general safeguards as provided as well as specific guidelines implemented by the 205th MI Cdr, FM 34-52, and the Commanding General, CJTF-7

FIGURE 3-2. *Interrogation poster from Abu Ghraib.*

medical personnel essentially vetted prisoners for interrogations that were designed in accord with the medical findings to include stress positions, sleep deprivation, isolation, dietary manipulation, threats, isolation, and so on. The findings from preinterrogation and postinterrogation exams were generally not kept with the prisoner's prison medical record. This double bookkeeping makes it impossible to know how carefully or how well the preinterrogation and postinterrogation physical examinations were done, and also makes it very easy to classify and thereby conceal signs of injuries that were noted after interrogations. Few of the MEDCOM (Medical Command) medical records declassified in response to an ACLU Freedom of Information Act lawsuit come from these interrogational medical records. The problem for investigators is exemplified by an investigation of an Abu Ghraib prisoner who claimed that a beating caused back pain. The physician told investigators that the prisoner, who was clearly paralyzed before the interrogation, suffered from a prior stroke and a painful back condition, spinal stenosis. The interrogator, however, said that the physician told him that the inmate was a "faker." The investigators did not review interrogation or medical records that might disclose what was actually communicated to the interrogators.[60]

Information from the preinterrogation medical exams had to be integrated into the design of interrogation plans. This process required a so-called biscuit.

General Miller created Behavioral Science Consultation Teams (BSCTs, or "biscuits") to work with the Intelligence Committees in Iraq and at Guantánamo. In his Iraq field assessment, he described the BSCTs' purpose thus: "These teams, comprised of operational behavioral psychologists and psychiatrists, are essential in developing integrated interrogation strategies and assessing interrogation intelligence production."[61] This statement must be translated in light of Secretary of Defense Rumsfeld's "counter resistance" interrogation directive: "Interrogations must . . . take into account . . . a detainee's emotional and physical strengths and weaknesses. . . . Interrogation approaches are designed to manipulate the detainee's emotions and weaknesses to gain his willing cooperation."[62] BSCTs played a central role in designing interrogation plans to exploit prisoners' psychological and physical weaknesses. Armed forces BSCTs are neither new nor, historically, sinister. The Defense Department has used them to evaluate soldiers' suitability for duty, develop ways to enhance troop cohesion, treat combat stress, and help veterans or POWs return to civilian life. The teams typically include mental health clinicians or behavioral scientists and some nonclinicians who are familiar with the military matter at hand. However, there was no precedent or policy for Miller's interrogational BSCTs.[63]

Abu Ghraib and Guantánamo BSCT personnel reviewed medical information relevant to the conduct of interrogations, performed psychological assessments, recommended physically and psychologically coercive interrogation plans, monitored and provided feedback during interrogations, and taught behavioral techniques to interrogators.[64,65] Abu Ghraib's BSCT was a subcommittee of the Military Intelligence Committee. For a time, it was chaired by Major Scott Uithol, a board-certified child psychiatrist, who in early 2004 also led the 113th Medical Company's Fitness Team at Camp Anaconda near Abu Ghraib, where he helped soldiers cope with combat stress.[66–68] Guantánamo's BSCT included a psychologist and psychiatrist, neither of whom were specialists in criminal investigative psychology. The BSCT's psychologist, Major John Leso, was a counseling psychologist with expertise assessing pilots' flight fitness.[69,70]

One of the most controversial of the BSCTs' powers was that of reviewing prisoners' medical records for material useful for selecting interrogation approaches.[71,72] Under Guantánamo's 2002 policy, medical personnel were obliged to give nonmedical personnel, including members of the BSCT, medical information relative to the "national security mission" upon request.[73,74] Guantánamo's Brigadier General Rick Baccus dismissed objections that this practice violated medical confidentiality and harmed the trust necessary to provide medical care. He said that medical records were routinely shared with intelligence personnel as physicians advised interrogators on whether prisoners were strong enough to withstand questioning.[75] General Miller simply denied to Red Cross officials that medical records were available to intelligence staff. The Red Cross protested the "integration of access to medical care within the system of coercion" to no avail.[76] Medical personnel in Iraq, in Afghanistan, and at Guantánamo confirmed that investigators had access to medical records, although most denied that military police or "other detention facility personnel" could see prisoners' medical records.[77] Given the shortage of clinicians at Abu Ghraib (see Chapter 5, "Neglect"), it seems improbable that they could have contributed detailed information to interrogators.

The medical clearance and BSCTs used clinical information for two purposes.

First, clinical examinations were used to "clear" prisoners for harsh interrogation plans. An intelligence officer at Camp Na'ma in Iraq complained that *every harsh interrogation was approved by the [commander] and the Medical* [emphasis in original] prior to its execution."[78] An Abu Ghraib guard, Sergeant Snider, succinctly said of the medically approved interrogation plans, "It became a problem for us because it took away from normal health and welfare for the inmates."[79]

Second, the BSCTs used medical and psychological information to develop a plan to break a prisoner's resistance to questioning. Clinicians at Guantánamo made records available to intelligence staff or met with BSCT personnel "to provide information about prisoners' mental health and vulnerabilities."[80] Such information included phobias (fear of the dark or of being alone) or medical conditions that could be exploited for "Fear Up Harsh," "We Know All," or "Environmental Manipulation" techniques. A military intelligence specialist in Iraq applied her background in psychology in a "special section" responsible for designing approaches to "interrogate those who could not be broken." She approved coercive interrogation plans involving sleep deprivation but vainly protested the use of dogs or nudity. She finally asked to be relieved of interrogation duties.[81] Steve Stefanowicz, a civilian "interrogator," testified that his requested interrogation plans could include sleep deprivation (four hours per day for three days then twelve hours' sleep and then repeated), sensory deprivation for up to seventy-two hours, "meal plans," isolating detainees "in the hole" for thirty days with a possible thirty-day extension, and shaving a detainee's beard or hair (to neutralize Muslims in the interrogation setting).[82] Behavioral clinicians reportedly micromanaged some interrogations; one anal Guantánamo psychiatrist suggested rationing toilet paper to seven sheets per day and limiting water for bathing.[83]

In November 2003, Colonel Pappas requested approval for the following interrogation plan for Abu Ghraib internee #15163, who was arrested deploying an explosive device in Baghdad:[84]

Detainee is at the point where he is resigned to the hope that Allah will see him through this episode in his life, therefore he feels no need to speak with interrogators. . . . Detainee needs to be put in a position where he will feel that the only option to get out of jail is to speak with interrogators.

Interrogators will establish control of detainee by allowing detainee to take this stance then implement a Fear Up Harsh approach. Interrogators will reinforce the fact that we have attempted to help him time and time again and that they are now putting it in Allah's hands. Interrogators will at a maximum throw tables, chairs, invade his personal space and continuously yell at the detainee. Interrogator will not physically touch or harm the detainees, will take all necessary precautions that all thrown objects are clear of the detainee and will not coerce the detainee in any way. If the detainee has not broken yet, interrogators will move into the segregation phase of the approach. Interrogators will coordinate with Military Police guards in the segregation area prior to initiation of this phase. . . . The MPs will put an empty sandbag onto the prisoner's head before moving him out of Vigilant B. . . . During transportation, the Fear Up Harsh approach will be continued, highlighting the Allah factor. . . . MP guards will take him into custody. MP working dogs will be present and barking during this phase.

Detainee will be strip searched by guards with the empty sandbag over his head for the safety of himself, prison guards, interrogators and other prisoners. Interrogators will wait outside the room while detainee is strip searched [by MPs]. Interrogators will watch from a distance while detainee is placed in the segregation cell. Detainee will be put on the adjusted sleep schedule (attached) for 72 hours. Interrogation will be conducted continuously during this 72 hour period. The approaches which will be used during this phase will include Fear Up Harsh, Pride Down, Ego Down, silence and loud music. Stress positions will also be used in accordance with CJTF-7 IROE [Interrogation Rules of Engagement] in order to intensify the approach.

It is reasonable to infer that a behavioral scientist helped design this proposal. At the time it was written, the Abu Ghraib BSCT was functional and psychological monitoring of interrogations was being done. The plan contains a psycho-cultural approach to exploiting the prisoner's religion. The reference to "not coercing" while applying "Fear Up Harsh," "Pride Down," "Ego Down," stress positions, barking dogs, strip searches, silence, a sandbag over the head, and loud noise to "break" the detainee in an environment where he has witnessed others being beaten is a tour-de-force of Orwellian language.

Interrogation Plans, such as proposed for inmate #15163, had to be approved before they could be implemented. Colonel Pappas, commander of the 205th Military Intelligence Brigade in Iraq, described the approval process this way, "Counter-resistance techniques had to fall within policy guidelines" and include "a sleep plan and medical standards. . . . [The] interrogation team then gives the interrogation plan directly to the MP guard that is going to work with Military Intelligence."[85] Once Colonel Pappas or General Sanchez approved a plan, copies went to the guards and to a "Tiger Team" consisting of an interrogator-translator and an intelligence analyst. Questioning focused on the organization and planning of the insurgency.[86,87] This orderly bureaucratic process often broke down in Iraq. Abu Ghraib had only one printer, and there were not enough filing cabinets to store interrogation plans. Interrogation data was not entered in computers and the software did not collate data for intelligence analysts. Delays in getting approvals of exceptional techniques were so common that the required approvals were sometimes not sought.[88–96]

The interrogation centers integrated the guards with the interrogators. Defense Secretary Rumsfeld directed that interrogation operations be "conducted in close cooperation with units detaining the individuals."[97] General Miller wrote that the prison environment must dedicate and train a detention guard force subordinate to the JIDC [Joint Interrogation and Debriefing Center] commander that sets the conditions for the successful interrogation and exploitation of internees/detainees. . . . Detention operations must be structured to ensure detention environment focuses the internee's confidence and attention on their interrogators. The MP detention staff should be an integrated element supporting the interrogation operations.[98]

General Sanchez's policy stated that interrogators should appear to "control all aspects of the interrogation to include the lighting, heating . . . as well as food, clothing and shelter given to security detainee."[99] At Mosul prison, the guards' general orders stated, "Firm control, coupled with mental stress, can greatly weaken a detainee's will. . . . The guard force will take all instructions from the Sergeant of the Guard . . . and interrogation team personnel [for] . . . providing appropriate mental stress on detainees."[100] The guards, for example, were allowed to do what was necessary to keep a prisoner awake during sleep management within the approved interrogation plan.[101] Sergeant Shannon Snider, an MP, described the process this way:

> We received guidance from Military Intelligence on altered diets, turning on and off the radio and sleep management. At first we didn't keep documentation and then we started getting everything in writing. . . . The requests were all laid out with times to do everything. . . . The requests were kept in the individual detainee's folder; we have a folder for each cell. . . . We tried to get limitations from Military Intelligence on what we could and could not do but never received any.[102]

This radical shift in Army policy blurred the chain of command in the prisons.[103] Previously, cellblock guards had provided "passive" prison security and had not been an "active" part of the interrogation process.[104] Military intelligence and the military police were jointly in charge; neither took responsibility for preventing abuses. As Major General Wojdakowski put it, "Clear cut chain of command does not exist in the prison. It is difficult to understand whom the Military Police work for, particularly in the MI [military intelligence] hold area."[105] Sergeant Javal Davis said that military intelligence personnel encouraged guards to abuse the detainees prior to interrogation, offering comments such as "Make sure he has a bad night," "Make sure he gets the treatment," "They're giving up good information finally," and "Keep up the good work."[106] Other MPs working at Abu Ghraib and in Afghanistan both reported and denied getting such urging.

MEDICAL MONITORING OF INTERROGATIONS

Medical monitoring of some harsh interrogations was policy and practice. Rumsfeld's interrogation directive required the "presence or availability of qualified medical personnel."[107] General Sanchez, the U.S. commander in Iraq, ordered that "interrogators will ensure that security internees are allowed adequate sleep; and that diets receive adequate food and water and cause no adverse medical or cultural effects. Where segregation is necessary, security internees must be monitored for adverse medical or psychological reactions."[108] Colonel Pappas, the military intelligence commander in Iraq, explained that a physician or psychiatrist, working "with the interrogators, would review all those people under a management plan and provide feedback as to whether they were being medically and physically taken care of."[109] The Interrogation Rules of Engagement poster that came from Afghanistan to Abu Ghraib include "Dietary Manip (monitored by med)" (see Figure 3.2).

Although few of the records describing interrogations have been declassified, investigative files, such as that concerning Al-Jamadi, confirm that clinicians were present during harsh interrogations. Guantánamo interrogators and officers reported that doctors observed interrogations from behind a mirror or were in the room during the interrogation.[110] In Iraq in 2004, a psychologist or Air Force physician attended interrogations that required psychological or medical supervision.[111–113] At Samarra, various soldiers offered sworn testimony about a particular interrogation.

A [Linguist—name redacted]: Specifically, regarding the screening interrogation of the Iraqi detainee known as [name redacted], I witnessed concern on the part of the primary interrogator toward preventing the detainee from going into a medical crisis as a result of the questioning. He stopped the questioning several times so that a medical professional could examine him and determine if he was still doing fine. All indications were that, aside from the stress of being captured and questioned, he was suffering no health crisis.

Q: During any interrogations did Staff Sergeant [name redacted] ever have to stop it because of medical problems?

A: I don't think so. The only one was [same inmate as above] but Staff Sergeant never stopped it. He only voiced concern that we ease up on the detainee so he could remain calm and keep his blood pressure down. . . .

A [Interrogator #1—name redacted]: All medications were put in the detainee's chest pocket.

A [Interrogator #2—name redacted]: [Name redacted] and I were the agents while [name redacted] sat in as the medic on standby. . . . Every time, maybe two or three times, the [detainee] showed any sign of difficulty, [co-interrogator] would take a break to allow [medic] to attend to him. . . . We took several breaks that night. The man was old and in the middle of the interrogation, we gathered up his pills (or medication) and gave it to him.[114]

At two locations in Iraq, a physician and a nurse reportedly either refused to administer, or witnessed the administration of, cough medicines or sedatives to persons undergoing interrogation.[115]

It is not possible for me to vet the interviews from human rights organizations and the media describing prisoners' reports of interrogation by psychiatrists. For example, Abdul Aziz Al-Swidi says that a psychiatrist actively interrogated him at Guantánamo.[116] BSCT clinicians had the authority to stop interrogations "on the spot," although one psychiatrist who admitted to having such authority paradoxically insisted that he never monitored one.[117]

Interrogation logs, detailing the medical monitoring of interrogations, remain classified—with one exception. This log was leaked from Guantánamo; excerpts were published by *Time,* and the Pentagon confirmed its authenticity.[118] In 2002, a BSCT psychologist, John Leso, monitored the interrogation of Mohammed al-Qahtani.[119] The fifty-day diary gives a detailed chronology of the application of isolation, sleep deprivation, humiliation, masking, head shaving, shackling, threatening with a dog, and so on. The log shows regular monitoring by medics, who, at one point, intravenously administered nearly three bags of medical saline while the prisoner was tied to a chair. When Mr. al-Qahtani asked to be allowed to urinate, he was told to urinate in his pants. He was treated twice, including at least one hospitalization, for a slow heart rate caused by hypothermia that was intentionally induced by means of air conditioning. Such heart disturbances can be very dangerous.[120,121] The physicians who aggressively treated this hypothermia, a condition unusual in tropical Cuba, returned him to the interrogators. It was FBI agents, not medical personnel, who complained about this life-threatening treatment.[122]

WITHHOLDING MEDICAL CARE DURING QUESTIONING

In December 2002, Defense Secretary Rumsfeld empowered Guantánamo interrogators to disapprove a prisoner's "medical visits of a non emergent nature."[123] This directive violates the Geneva Convention Relative to the Treatment of Prisoners of War: "Prisoners of war may not be prevented from presenting themselves to the medical authorities for examination." A month later, on the advice of legal counsel, Rumsfeld revoked this order.[124]

Nevertheless, the practice of punitive denial of treatment apparently continued throughout the prison system. In Pakistan, Abu Zubaydah, a senior Al Qaeda official, was shot in the chest, groin, and thigh during his capture in March 2002. A month later, Secretary Rumsfeld announced, "We have him. He is under U.S. control. We are responsible for him. . . . He is receiving medical care and we intend to get every single thing out of him to try to prevent terrorist acts in the future."[125] Several sources report that interrogators withheld painkillers and may have administered mind-altering drugs to procure information during his interrogation.[126–128] In Afghanistan, a sergeant was accused of denying medical care to the badly beaten Dilawar, whose death will be discussed in the next chapter. In Iraq, a prisoner at Tikrit testified to Army investigators that he was not given an opportunity to see a doctor for injuries suffered during interrogation. A letter of reprimand appears to have been written.[129] Army investigators reviewed a video showing a prisoner with bound wrists lying on the ground near a checkpoint. Entry and exit gunshot wounds are visible. While the soldiers discuss whether to summon medical care, one soldier tells the moaning prisoner to "shut up" and kicks him in the face or upper chest. A soldier who was present during the videotaping later joked that "[we] weren't in any hurry to call the medics," adding that he "thought the dude eventually died."[130]

A recently filed civil lawsuit and an FBI memo describe four prisoners, three at Guantánamo and one apparently in Afghanistan, who were denied a prosthetic limb, antibiotics for festering wounds (two cases), and treatment for constipation until they cooperated with interrogators.[131] An FBI memo tells of a prisoner, arrested in Afghanistan, who was denied treatment for a gunshot wound while he was tortured for at least three days before being taken to a hospital for treatment. During torture, he fabricated statements to get the mistreatment to abate.[132] A Guantánamo prisoner told an FBI agent a similar story.[133] At Guantánamo Bay, a psychology technician complained to the officer in charge about the officer's refusal to allow a prisoner to receive a medical evaluation of his back pain. The officer answered, "Listen, bitch, I run this cellblock the way I see fit. If I think a detainee is complaining about back pain just to get to walk across the camp to the medical clinic one sunny afternoon, then I'm not going to put it in my log. Now leave my block and next time stay in your lane."[134] Another Guantánamo interrogator, who had read a prisoner's medical files, asked for medical treatment of his eyes; his commander replied, "Fuck him. He should have gotten the medical help before he went on Jihad."[135]

THE DEFENSE DEPARTMENT RESPONDS

Public criticism of clinical assistance with harsh interrogations mounted throughout the summer of 2004. Initially, the Defense Department entirely denied reporters' and medical writers' allegations of abuses or improper procedures. It insisted that medical personnel were only "on hand," rather than overseeing the design or monitoring of interrogations, and that intelligence personnel who were not clinicians stopped interrogations if medical care was needed.[136,137] The assistant secretary of defense for health, William Winkenwerder, Jr., M.D., rejected the allegation that medical personnel had any say in setting the severity of interrogations or were advised "to look the other way" as prisoners were mistreated. He stated, "We have no evidence of maltreatment by physicians, or of physicians participating in torture or torturous activity. We just do not have evidence of that. . . . We always expect a physician to behave ethically in any circumstance."[138] Dr. Winkenwerder and medical commanders jointly claimed, "Military medical personnel are obliged to report to the proper authorities when they suspect that a prisoner is being mistreated or harmed at any time, including during interrogation."[139] As late as July 2005, the Army Surgeon General, Lieutenant General Kevin Kiley, was still insisting, "We found no evidence that . . . there was a passing of clinical information that would be used in a detrimental way to torture."[140] However, Dr. Kiley's investigators did not even ask psychologists to describe the information or recommendations that they provided to interrogators.

David Tornberg, M.D., the Defense Department's deputy assistant secretary for health, contradicted Surgeon General Kiley and said that it was proper to use clinicians and medical records for interrogations. Indeed he argued, interrogators "could not conduct their job without that info." He went on to say that intelligence officers had complete freedom to collect, transfer, and use "military relevant" clinical information because, as he bluntly put it, there was "no doctor-patient relationship" for such prisoners.[141]

Dr. Winkenwerder claimed that inmates of U.S. federal prisons do "not have a complete and absolute right to privacy of medical information." Although the federal Bureau of Prisons does permit the gathering of medical evidence, such as DNA samples, without a prisoner's consent and does not protect the privacy of medical information that threatens prison security, prisoners' medical records may not be requisitioned for use in coercive interrogation.[142]

Bowing to public pressure, the Pentagon cosmetically revised its clinical confidentiality policy in June 2005. The new policy accepted Dr. Tornberg's novel proposal that there was one set of ethics for clinicians who treated prisoners and another set for those who worked with interrogators.[143,144] Accordingly, the revised policy barred treating clinicians from "actively solicit[ing] information from detainees for purposes other than health care purposes," while it empowered mental health specialists working with interrogators to breach confidentiality for "any lawful . . . intelligence or national security related activity."[145] Physicians for Human Rights has detailed how the Defense Department's revised policy for interrogational clinicians extensively conflicts with the UN Principles of Medical Ethics of 1982.[146] The current Defense Department policy is that psychiatrists and physicians may serve on the BSCTs.[147,148]

Vice Admiral Albert Church's 2005 investigation of prisons in Afghanistan, in Iraq, and at Guantánamo Bay found that "behavioral science personnel observe interrogations, assess detainee behavior and motivations, review interrogation techniques, and offer advice to interrogators"; but, the admiral said, they were not "permitted access to detainee medical records for the purposes of developing interrogation strategies." He then muddied the waters:

> While access to medical information was carefully controlled at Guantanamo, we found in Afghanistan and Iraq that interrogators sometimes had easy access to such information. Nevertheless, we found no instances where detainee medical information had been inappropriately used during interrogations and, in most situations, interrogators had little interest in detainee medical information even when they had unfettered access to it.

The classified appendices to Church's investigation may reveal how diligently his investigators searched for the inappropriate use of medical information.

Admiral Church accepted the distinction drawn by Drs. Winkenwerder and Tornberg between the ethical obligations of clinicians who treated prisoners as patients, and the obligations of those working with interrogators. Although he insisted that the medical and behavioral science personnel working with interrogators "were not involved in providing medical care," he justified communications between treating clinicians and interrogational clinicians with a vague proposal that is open to abusive interpretation:

> Interrogators often have legitimate reasons for inquiring into detainees' medical status. For example, interrogators need to be able to verify whether detainees are being truthful when they claim that interrogations should be restricted on medical grounds. Granting interrogators unfettered access to detainee medical records, however, raises the problem that detainees' medical information could be inappropriately exploited during interrogations.

Admiral Church said that policies and practices for engaging medical staff in interrogations had evolved in an ad hoc process with little deliberation, and he concluded: "A policy review is needed to address the status of medical personnel (such as behavioral scientists supporting interrogators) who do not participate in patient care."[149]

DISCUSSION

Interrogation that uses physical or psychological stress is not a therapeutic medical procedure. Substituting mind-altering drugs for hot irons does not move interrogation into the ambit of health care, any more than death by means of Dr. Louis's decapitator constituted surgery because it did not involve breaking a person on the wheel. Simply put, health professionals are accountable for the health of their patients, regardless of the fact of imprisonment. Many statements by the UN, international medical and human rights organizations, and American medical societies directly and unambiguously bar physicians, nurses, and other health personnel from participating in the design, application, or monitoring of coercive, harsh, inhumane, or stressful interrogations. The U.S. armed forces have ignored these standards. The use of clinicians to clear or monitor persons for harsh or coercive interrogation violates numerous codes of medical ethics. As the American College of Physicians succinctly puts it,

> Under no circumstances is it ethical for a physician to be used as an instrument of government to weaken the physical or mental resistance of a human being, nor should a physician participate in or tolerate cruel or unusual punishment or disciplinary activities beyond those permitted by the United Nations Standard Minimum Rules for the Treatment of Prisoners.
>
> ... The doctor's fundamental role is to alleviate the distress of his or her fellow men, and no motive whether personal, collective or political shall prevail against this higher purpose.

The American Medical Association, the International Council of Nurses, the World Medical Association, the UN in its Principles of Medical Ethics, and all the other medical codes and societies listed in the bibliography concur.

Within the primary obligation to promote a person's well-being, distinctions are possible to allow behavioral scientists, psychologists, or psychiatrists to work with forensic interviews. It is one thing for such clinicians to train an interrogator in rapport-building skill and cross-cultural communication. It is quite another to use psychological, medical, and cultural information (especially when obtained in a clinical encounter) to degrade, frighten, or inflict physical distress on a person in order to coerce information from that person. It is a duty to monitor a prisoner's health; it is an abuse to monitor a prisoner so that the interrogator has information to increase or decrease the degree of physical or psychic stress.

Medical professionals cooperated with all phases of coercive interrogation in Iraq, at Guantánamo, and in Afghanistan. Some provided information from medical records, clinical interviews, and medical examinations to interrogators for use in designing interrogation plans. Some worked with or on Behavioral Science Consultation Teams that recommended ways to break down prisoners. Behavioral scientists used insights from cross-cultural psychology to degrade and demoralize prisoners. Some clinicians monitored interrogations to manage the risks of health-endangering techniques. There is no difference between the medic who monitored the old man's blood pressure and heart rate during the interrogation in Samarra and the "doctor" who measured the same vital signs of a Venezuelan prisoner, occasionally allowing him "a little rest" before the abuse resumed.[150]

In such acts, clinicians betrayed the duties of the healing profession and the well-being of their imprisoned patients. By damaging prisoners' trust in the medical system, clinicians made prisoners less likely to confide health concerns for the sake of their own medical care and, potentially, for the early discovery of contagious diseases, such as tuberculosis, which could spread throughout the prison staff and inmate population.[151]

Medical ethics codes condemn any medical involvement with the administration of punishments. As the British Medical Association pointedly stated twenty years ago, with respect to the abuse of Irish Republican Army prisoners, "Any diet so restricted that medical monitoring is necessary is inhuman, and no doctor should be associated with it."[152] We may extend the implication to any treatment of prisoners.

CHAPTER 4

HOMICIDE

DILAWAR WAS A TWENTY-TWO-YEAR-OLD FARMER AND TAXI DRIVER, whom American soldiers tortured to death over five days at Bagram Collection Point in Afghanistan in December 2002.[1,2] When the soldiers pulled a sandbag over his head, Dilawar complained that he could not breathe. He was then shackled and suspended from his arms for hours, denied water, and beaten so severely that his legs would have been amputated had he survived. When he was beaten with a baton, he would cry "Allah, Allah!," which guards found so amusing that they beat him some more just to hear him cry. During his final interrogation, soldiers told the delirious, injured prisoner that he would get medical attention after the session. Instead, he was returned to a cell and chained to the ceiling. Several hours later, a physician found him dead. By then, the interrogators had concluded that Dilawar was innocent and had simply been picked up after driving his new taxi by the wrong place at the wrong time.

Dilawar's death was predictable and preventable. The counterintelligence team was inexperienced; only two of its thirteen soldiers had ever conducted interrogations before arriving in Afghanistan. The officers knew that President Bush and Secretary Rumsfeld had ruled that the Geneva Conventions did not apply to Afghanistan. The interrogation policies were unclear. The base commander had ignored Red Cross protests about the treatment of prisoners, including the practice of suspending them. Army and intelligence officers who knew of the ongoing pattern of abuses at the Bagram facility did not intervene to stop them. In fact, another prisoner, Habibullah, had died at the same facility under similar circumstances six days before Dilawar's death.[3,4]

An autopsy on December 13 found that Dilawar's death was a homicide, caused by extensive and severe "blunt force injuries to lower extremities complicating coronary artery disease" (inexplicably, "coronary artery disease" is typed on the death certificate in a different font).[5] The Pentagon reported that the prisoner died of natural causes. Later, a coroner testified that Dilawar's legs were "pulpified" and that the body looked as if it had been "run over by a truck." Soldiers delivered the body and an English-language death certificate to his wife and two daughters in January 2003. The family could not read English.

In February, General Daniel McNeil, the commander of U.S. forces in Afghanistan, told reporters that Dilawar died of natural causes and that 85 percent of his coronary artery was obstructed. He said that he had "no indication" that Dilawar had been injured in prison; later, he said that the prisoner had been injured before arriving at Bagram and went on to assert, "We are not chaining people to the ceilings." General Daniel McNeil was evidently familiar with Dilawar's autopsy, which had found that a coronary artery was 70 percent to 80 percent occluded even though that heart disease did not cause his death.[6] The Office of the Armed Forces Medical Examiner, which had done the autopsy, did not contradict General McNeil's statements and did not release the death certificate or autopsy report.

Later in February, reporters went to Dilawar's village and located his family, who had the copy of the death certificate stating that Dilawar had died of homicidal injuries. The reporters confronted General McNeil with the death certificate that had been given to the family and asked him to explain why he had told reporters that Dilawar died a natural death of heart disease. General McNeil said that he always gave press the "best information available to him."[7]

Dilawar has two or three death certificates. The family's certificate, finalized on December 13, 2002, fills in a box captioned "Circumstances Surrounding Death Due to External Causes" with "Decedent was found unresponsive in his cell while in custody."[8] A year and a half after the death, the Pentagon released another death certificate, finalized on May 20, 2004, that does not describe the circumstances in which the body was found.[9] The Defense Department released yet another death cer-

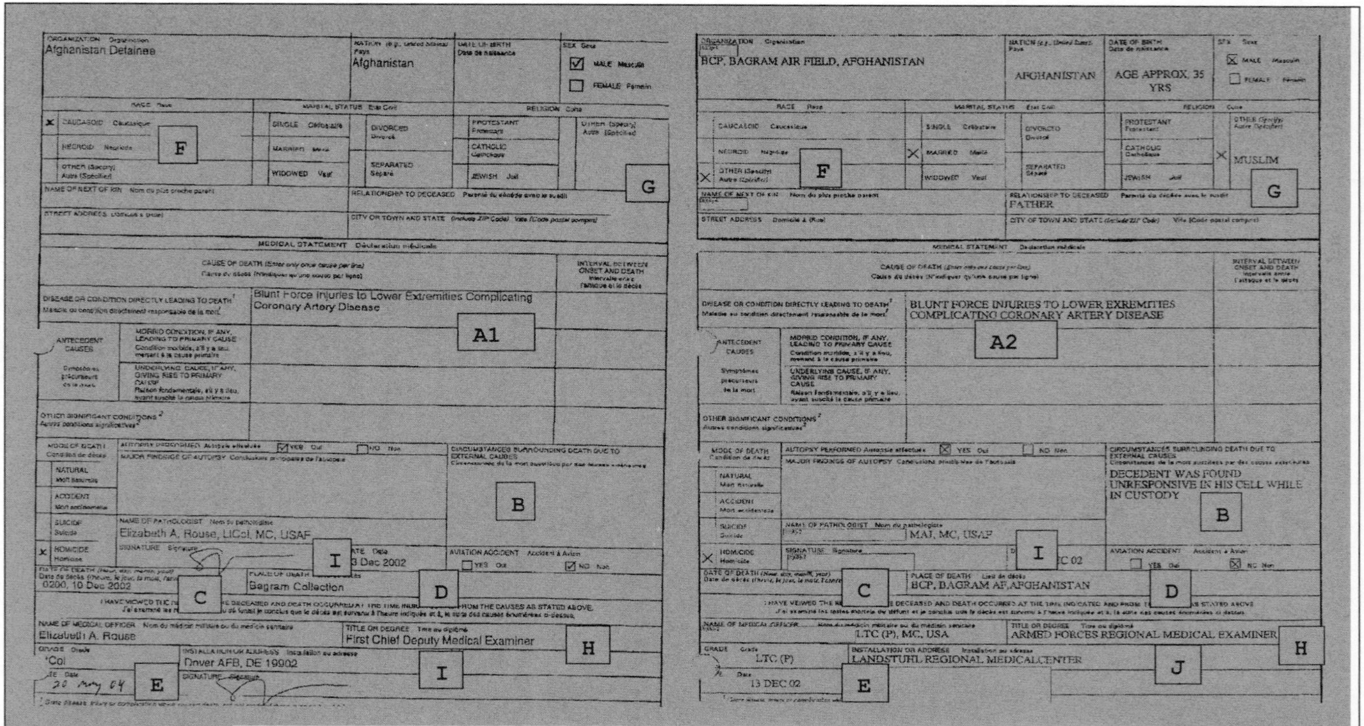

FIGURE 4.1. Dilawar's two death certificates.

A1: Two-font cause of death   D: Location of death   H: Title of examiner

A2: One-font cause of death   E: Date of death   I: Signature of examiner

B: Circumstances of death   F: Race   J: Location of certification of

C: Date of death   G: Religion   death

tificate in April 2005.[10] That document, dated December 2002, may be the one given to the family. It includes the description of the death's discovery and adds Dilawar's age and religion, but omits the date of death and changes the title and address of the pathologist.

Dilawar is not the only prisoner who died a violent death for whom there exists more than one death certificate. The Pentagon has released two differing death certificates for Fahin Ali Gumaa, who died of multiple gunshot wounds. One certificate was finalized May 21, 2004, just before a Pentagon press conference, and the other was finalized June 2, 2004, after the press conference.[11] The usual rule for death certificates is "one per customer."

Army criminal investigators waited sixteen months to begin investigating Dilawar's death. They found probable cause to charge twenty-seven soldiers with various roles in causing and concealing the death, including a charge of withholding medical care. No one was charged with murder. Five of the fifteen who were prosecuted have pleaded guilty to assault and other crimes. The harshest punishment received was five months in a military prison. One soldier was convicted of maiming, assault, maltreatment, and making a false statement; he was demoted and honorably discharged. Dilawar left a widow and two-year-old daughter. One of his brothers, Shahpoor, reacted to the sentences this way: "I am angry with them, but this was the will of God. God is great, and God will punish them."[12] Vice Admiral Church identified Dilawar's death as one in which medical personnel might have tried to conceal the abuse of a prisoner.[13]

PRISONERS TORTURED TO DEATH

Nineteen prisoners are known to have died of beatings, asphyxiation, or being suspended by American soldiers or intelligence officials.[14] These men died at Asadabad, Bagram, and Gardez in Afghanistan and at Abu Ghraib, Camp Bucca, Camp Whitehorse, Basra, Mosul, Tikrit, and another unidentified facility in Iraq.

The figure of nineteen deaths from torture does not include all prisoners whose deaths were homicides, or all prisoners who died by torture. It does not include criminal homicides that took place on the battlefield or in the interval between capture and imprisonment. It does not include prisoners who died of injuries wantonly inflicted by Afghan or Iraqi soldiers working with U.S. forces, even when such a badly beaten prisoner was turned over to U.S. authorities before dying in U.S. custody.[15] It does not include homicides by torture that were committed by British soldiers, such as the deaths of Baha Mousa and Kifah Taha, listed in the table at the end of this chapter. It undoubtedly fails to include some homicides of "ghost prisoners," such as Al-Jamadi, whose death was described in the preceding chapter—people who were secretly imprisoned by U.S. intelligence agencies. It does not include homicides among the deaths that were not investigated or that were only superficially investigated, or where the investigations were preempted by base commanders. It does not include cases where a homicide was misattributed to natural causes. It does not include homicides among the prisoners who have likely died after U.S. authorities sent them to be interrogated in torturing countries such as Uzbekistan. It does not include at least twenty "justified" shootings of "rioting" prisoners. (For example, in September 2003, a Red Cross observer witnessed a guard shooting a Camp Bucca prisoner through the chest and wrote: "The shooting showed a clear disregard for human life and security of the persons deprived of their liberty." The Army concluded that the shooting was justifiable.[16] Major General Antonio Taguba, who conducted the Army's first investigation of the Abu Ghraib scandal, noted similar incidents.[17]) It does not include prisoners who died of medical neglect or after being needlessly and illegally exposed to mortar and sniper attacks on prisons (see Chapter 5, "Neglect") A map of the topography of "substantiated" criminal homicides, justified homicides, and unsubstantiated-as-homicide prisoners' deaths looks like this.

Substantiated criminal homicide (e.g., death from torture)

Substantiated justified homicide (e.g., shooting of rioting prisoner)

Homicide unsubstantiated because of obstructed investigation (e.g., local commander obstructs investigation, or prisoner dies after rendition to a torturing country, or unregistered prisoner dies in small base prison, or unregistered prisoner dies in intelligence agency custody)

Unrecognized homicide (e.g., death mistakenly attributed to natural causes)

MEDICAL INVESTIGATIONS OF PRISONERS' DEATHS

The Armed Forces Institute of Pathology is responsible for determining the cause of death of a prisoner in U.S. facilities in Iraq, in Afghanistan, and at Guantánamo Bay.[18,19] In 1996, it created the Office of the Armed Forces Medical Examiner (AFME) to conduct autopsies of soldiers and civilians (including prisoners) who died while in the armed forces or under their jurisdiction. In 2002, budget cutbacks left the AFME with only two forensic pathologists; by 2004, it had thirteen.[20]

Armed forces medical examiners' autopsy reports and death certificates as well as Army and Navy criminal investigation reports show that pathologists often did not seem to have been given information ordinarily available to pathologists. A pathologist bases a determination of cause of death on more than an autopsy. An autopsy, or necropsy, entails inspecting and dissecting a body, examining organs, performing toxicology and chemical tests, and looking at tissues with a microscope or sometimes with X rays. The pathologist correlates the autopsy findings with information from medical records, accounts of the events preceding the death, and a description of the circumstances in which the body was found. As noted in the preceding chapter on interrogations, preinterrogation and postinterrogation medical examinations, if conducted at all, were kept in classified intelligence files separate from regular medical records. Chapter 5, "Neglect," will show that even these regular medical records were haphazardly kept and often lost in Iraq and Afghanistan. Even when clinical records and death scene descriptions existed, pathologists' and field investigators' reports show mostly one-way communication between forensic pathologists and Army or Navy criminal investigators. Pathologists performed autopsies and forwarded their findings and death certificates to investigators who did the event analysis. In other words, the pathologists often had to determine the cause of death without on-site investigative findings. For example, the physical findings at autopsy of a person who dies of suffocation, a common cause of death among recognized prisoner homicides, can be very subtle. A pathologist must know whether the prisoner had a hood over his head or was gagged, suspended, or bound in a manner that could prevent the chest from expanding and the victim from inhaling. Information to include or exclude such possibilities is absent from many of the autopsy reports.

The Office of the Armed Forces Medical Examiner was inadequately prepared to investigate deaths of prisoners who may have died of torture. Its pathologists had published little on forensic pathology. They were not known for having special expertise in investigating or documenting the injuries of persons who died under torture. There is no evidence that they used a special protocol for conducting autopsies on prisoners who may have died from torture. It does not even appear that they were familiar with protocols such as the "Manual on the Investigation of Torture and Other Cruel, Inhuman, or Degrading Treatment," a guide, endorsed by the UN and the World Medical Association, for physicians who examine bodies for signs of death by torture.[21] That manual recommends that pathologists inspect bodies for signs of beatings, thermal and chemical burns, visible and invisible fractures, signs of the use of tight ligatures around the penis or extremities, suffocation, brain damage, suspension tears to ligaments or muscles or nerves, and anal or vaginal penetration. The AFME autopsies often failed to look for injuries to bones or ligaments or for signs of sexual abuse. For example, Mr. Al-Jamadi (discussed in Chapter 3) died while being suspended by his arms, which had been tied together and lifted up behind his back. Witnesses reported that his shoulders were twisted and protruding out of their sockets, but the pathologist did not even record an examination of the shoulders for dislocation or for tearing of the ligaments and nerves of the upper arms.

DEATH CERTIFICATES

A death certificate is the legal record of a person's death. This document identifies the decedent by name and birthday. It names the next of kin and the decedent's religion so that relatives can be notified and so that remains are handled with respect for the decedent's culture. It notes the time, place, and cause of death. Finally, it records a physician's conclusion as to whether that cause of death was "natural" or a result of an "accident," "suicide," or "homicide." That conclusion sets the stage for legal action. If the death was due to homicide, investigators and a prosecutor must determine whether the homicide was premeditated, impulsive, unintended, or justifiable. If the death resulted from an accident, was criminal negligence involved? Most physicians know the basics of completing the deceptively simple death certificate. A medical examiner's or forensic pathologist's job is to complete a death certificate in difficult circumstances.

On May 21, 2004, the Defense Department held a press conference to address concerns about homicides and natural deaths of prisoners in Iraq and Afghanistan.[22] It distributed the biographies of the senior officials who were giving the briefing to a large group of reporters, who obsequiously agreed not to release the names of the two senior Defense Department spokespersons. The Pentagon proposed that these spokespersons be called "senior military official" and "senior defense official." The reporters won permission to call them "senior military official" and "senior department medical official." The obfuscation over names only set the stage for a bizarre briefing.

The purpose of the briefing was to discuss thirty death investigations concerning prisoners, who were not named. Nine of the cases were still under active investigation. Twenty-three death certificates were given to the press, but the officials would not say if these were deaths that were or had been under investigation or some other deaths.[23,24]

The reporters soon went from baffled to hostile. The officers would not say how many of the cases under investigation were from Iraq or Afghanistan. They dodged questions about the location and circumstances of the deaths, even when reporters simply asked them to confirm information from other reliable sources. Finally, an exasperated reporter asked:

Reporter: Sir, rather than us playing "find the peanut" . . . is it possible for you to go though any subset of these, perhaps the nine [cases under active investigation], and tell us what date it happened and as much detail as you can about it?

Senior Military Official: What I can tell you on the nine—I think what I can tell you safely on the nine, because they're ongoing investigations—and really it was already asked. You know, the time frame goes from December of '02 to present.

The twenty-three death certificates released at the press conference did not comply with accepted medical practice. Most did not contain information required by the Geneva Convention: surname, first name(s); rank, army, regimental, serial number (these four did apply to prisoners from the Iraqi military); birth date; date, place, and cause of death; date, place, and location of burial. Thirteen did not note the date of birth, a vital statistic that should have been obtained at the time of imprisonment and which is useful for evaluating the conclusion that many prisoners died of heart attacks. None of them recorded the names of next of kin, which were also supposed to have been collected at the time of imprisonment. None gave the disposition of the remains. Many did not specify where the death occurred: four simply said "Iraq," whereas standard practice would record the name of the prison. With rare exceptions, pathologists did not complete the sections headed "Other Significant Conditions," "Major Autopsy Findings," and "Circumstances Surrounding Death Due to External Causes." Given that half of the deaths were caused by abuse, it is hard to believe that prisoners who died of "natural causes" did not have noteworthy trauma at autopsy.

The press conference's death certificates also showed that the Defense Department was improperly withholding the public release of prisoners' death certificates. Normally, death certificates are completed within a few days or weeks after a death or autopsy. The Army's standard is to complete a death certificate within two weeks of an autopsy. Seventeen of the twenty-three death certificates released at the May 2004 press conference were finalized in the nine days before the briefing although the deaths had occurred months or years earlier. The delay in the release of the death certificates was produced by simply having the pathologists delay the completion of their work.

In several instances, the Defense Department pathologist affixed his or her preliminary and final signatures to multiple certificates at a single sitting shortly before the press conference. For example, Major Michael E.

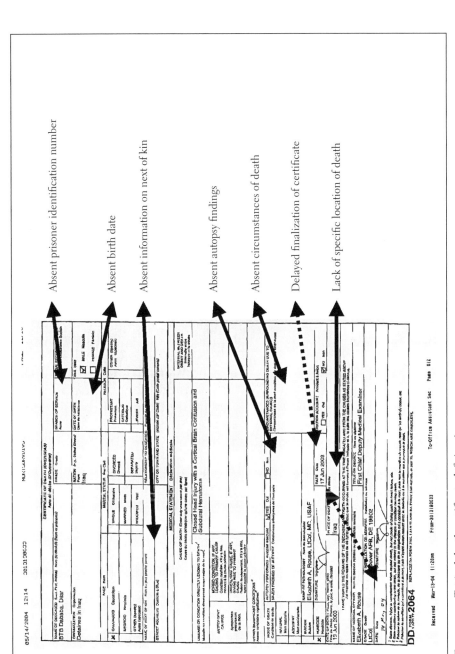

FIGURE 4.2. Typical death-certificate deficiencies.

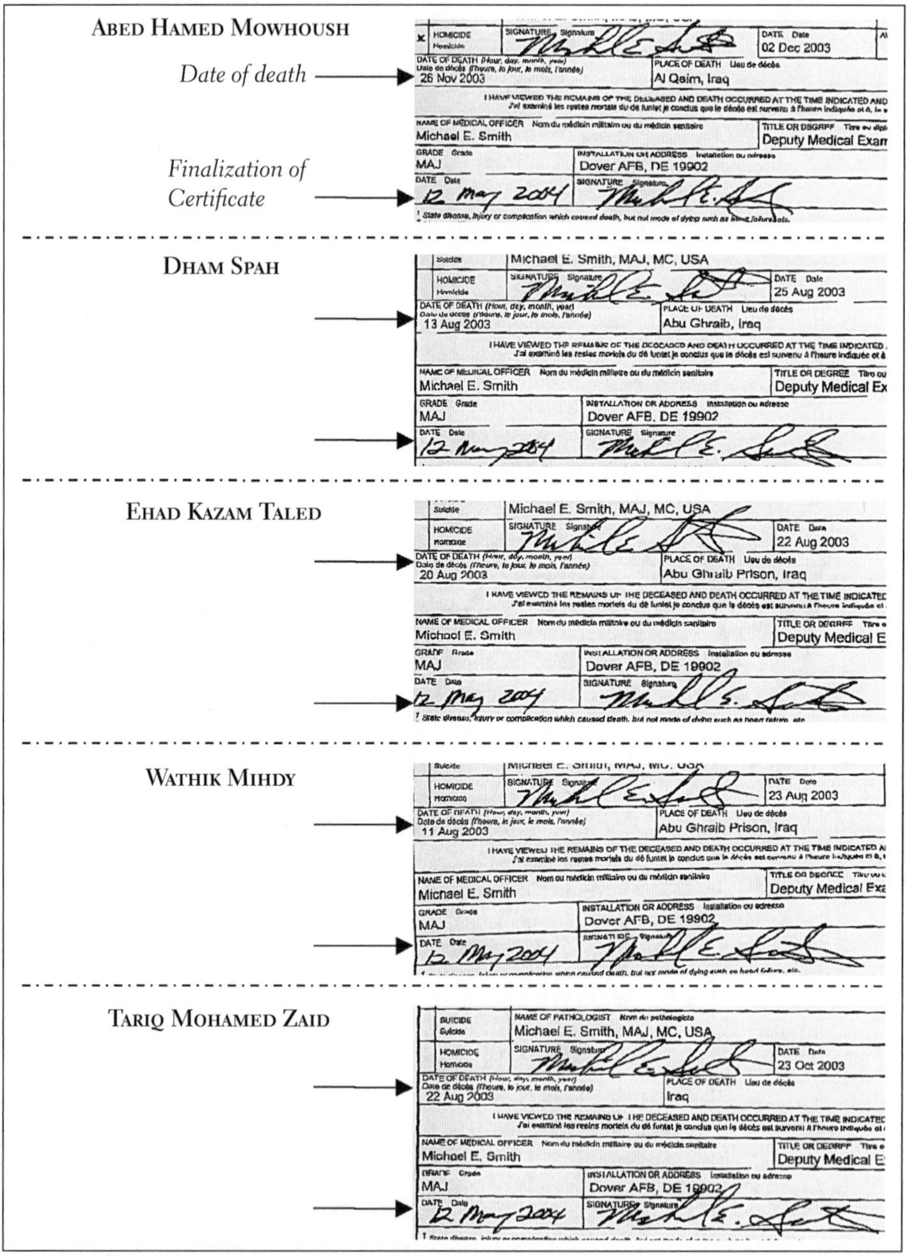

FIGURE 4.3. *Major Michael Smith's delayed death-certificate signatures.*

Smith finalized five death certificates on May 12, 2004, nine days before the Pentagon press conference where they were released. Figure 4.3 shows that he apparently used one pen and hand stroke for his initial and finalization signatures on August 22, 23, and 25 and on October 23 and December 2, 2003, and on May 12, 2004.[25–29] A similar pattern is seen on death certificates signed by Colonel Eric Berg, Lieutenant Colonel Elizabeth Rouse, and Major Louis Finelli. James Caruso also did the same on the three death certificates he prepared; he even signed one on behalf of a pathologist named Jerry Hodges, on May 13, 2004.

"OBSTRUCTED INVESTIGATIONS"

Army and intelligence officials' power to obstruct or delay investigations of deaths in Iraq and Afghanistan contributed to investigators' inability to "substantiate" some homicides. A prisoner at Husaybah prison in Iraq attempted to escape twenty times in thirty-six hours before reportedly throwing himself out of a window and dying of "head trauma." That he was able to throw himself out a window, given the routine restraint of uncooperative prisoners, beggars belief. The camp commander delayed reporting the death. A cursory investigation, conducted more than a month after the body had been buried near the prison, was inconclusive.[30] A Tikrit commander delayed an investigation until after he had administratively preempted the possibility of prosecuting an indicted soldier who shot and killed Obeed Hethere Radad.[31–33] Mohammed Khan died in Camp Salerno in Afghanistan; his family says the body bore signs of torture. Colonel Gary Cheeks told a reporter that Khan died of a snakebite, adding, "You could go on for ages with a 'he said, she said.' You have to take my word for it."[34] Afghanistan has two species of poisonous snakes. The McMahon's viper is very rarely seen; the Levant viper stays away from settlements. An autopsy was not done.

In 2004, at Camp Cropper, an Iraq prison where many inmates were abused, at least three investigations were closed without autopsies. Also at Camp Cropper, Mohammad Munim al-Izmerly died shortly after his family visited him in prison in early 2004. They found him to be in good health. After his death, the body was held for more than two weeks, during which time camp officials failed to notify either Army criminal investigators or al-Izmerly's family of the death. U.S. soldiers finally left the body at a Baghdad hospital along with a death certificate saying that he had died of a "sudden brainstem compression." The family commissioned an autopsy by the director of the hospital's pathology service, who found that a massive blow to al-Izmerly's head had caused the brain injury.[35] A press report tells of two other Camp Cropper prisoners who died under unusual circumstances but whose bodies were not autopsied.[36] One died after he "fell out of bed and struck his head. A CAT scan showed intracranial trauma and signs of previous head injuries." The second was found "unresponsive by guards." Camp officers claimed that the body "did not exhibit any signs of abuse or foul play" and did not inform Army investigators of the death.

It was very difficult to investigate or declassify information about the deaths of CIA prisoners. Mr. Hadi Abdul Hussain Hasson was a ghost prisoner at Camp Bucca in Iraq. He was captured on an unknown date in the spring of 2003. Army investigators learned of his death on July 27, 2004. The investigator dryly notes, "Due to inadequate record keeping, this office could only estimate that Mr. Hasson possibly died between April–Sept 03." Mr. Hasson's name was absent from the camp roster, military intelligence notes, medical records, and autopsy reports; this absence is a hallmark of ghost prisoners, imprisoned under the authority of the CIA. Army investigators were not able to substantiate a criminal homicide but they did find a note referring to a complaint lodged soon after Mr. Hasson's imprisonment: "Preliminary investigation has revealed the following detainees have alleged they were abused while in Coalition custody . . . Hussain Hasson."[37] The Army Surgeon General spoke with an unidentified clinician who complained that in two cases,

he was pressured by OGA ["Other Government Agencies," jargon that usually refers to the CIA] into filling out death certificates on Iraqi Detainees. Stated he was not given the opportunity to examine the dead. Causes of death were later found to be inaccurate. CID [Criminal Investigation Division] investigated.[38]

Apparently, this investigation has not been declassified.

In addition to ghost detainees, military patrols held unregistered prisoners in small forward bases. Such prisoners could disappear. The *Los Angeles Times* uncovered the case of Jamal Naseer, who was picked up by U.S. Special Forces in Afghanistan in March 2003. Mr. Naseer was held in a small, overcrowded detention cell at Gardez. This facility did not register its prisoners and was closed to Red Cross monitors. No medical personnel visited Naseer during the seventeen days over which he was beaten. Men arrested with Mr. Naseer were beaten, kicked, whipped, slammed against the wall, and immersed in cold water. Their toenails either fell off or were torn off. Eyewitnesses saw Mr. Naseer falling to the ground, suffering a seizure, and then dying. He was bleeding from his ear. That clinical history suggests that he died of a basilar skull fracture caused by severe head trauma. Four months later, the Pentagon omitted his death from a list of thirty-nine prisoner deaths. In fact, the Pentagon claimed that it did not even know of his case until the Crimes of War Project told them of the matter.[39] Six months after Mr. Naseer's death, Human Rights Watch reported that the Army had opened an inquiry; nothing further is known.[40] Nasrat Mohammad "Amer" Abed al-Latif also disappeared after being taken into custody. The twenty-three-year-old Iraqi physics student was shot during a raid on his house by armed men in plainclothes who appeared to be U.S. nationals. His father and two brothers were detained for five days. Soldiers told the family that they had taken the injured Amer to a medical facility, where he had died, and that his body would be returned to them. Amnesty International reports that neither his body nor any records of his imprisonment and care can be found.[41]

It is possible that reports of the deaths of women and children prisoners are being suppressed, just as photographs of sexual poses of women prisoners at Abu Ghraib have been withheld from the public. The Defense Department has not released the death certificate or autopsy of a child known to have died of tuberculosis at Camp Cropper. That child's death is mentioned only in an aside in a footnote commenting on another case in the report of an Army investigation.[42] Similarly, a one-page summary of legal actions refers to a legal investigation of the death of an Iraqi woman in an incident involving the 4th Engineering Battalion.[43] No death certificate, autopsy report, or other record of that death exists.

A final category of invisible prisoners comprises those whom the CIA has sent to countries that practice torture. The fates of nearly all of the hundreds of persons subjected to these irregular extraditions are unknown.[44] The United States is responsible for any mistreatment or homicides of such prisoners; however, the Army Surgeon General statements carefully avoid any claim of responsibility for the well-being or death investigations of such prisoners.[45]

"NATURAL DEATHS"

It is neither surprising, nor entirely avoidable, that some homicides are misclassified as natural deaths. Many death certificates assert that prisoners died "natural" deaths from heart attacks. The forensic investigators do not seem to explore the relationship between mistreatment and lethal heart attacks caused by stress. Scientific research shows that arrest, threats, beatings, fear, and police interrogation can all cause "homicide by heart attack," or life-threatening heart failure. People with preexisting heart disease, dehydration, hyperthermia, or exhaustion are especially at risk.[46–50] Some "natural" heart attacks have followed harsh treatment during arrest. A typically sketchy Army report notes,

> Detainee Death during weekend combat. During a jointly conducted, Army led raid this past weekend of a house in Iraq . . . an Iraqi who was detained and "zip-locked" [flexi-cuffed with plastic bands tying his wrists together] died while in custody. Preliminary information is that the detainee died from an apparent heart attack.[51]

Human rights organizations have described similar events. For example, Human Rights Watch reports that soldiers detained Sher Mohammad Khan in Afghanistan in September 2004. Shortly thereafter, his bruised body was given to his family. Military officials told journalists that he had died of a heart attack within hours of being taken into custody. No investigative record, autopsy, or death certificate is available.[52] The Christian Peacemaker Team describes a similar event that also suggests stress-induced heart attack. On December 21, 2003, soldiers burst into the home of Mehadi Al Jamal, a retired land surveyor who had lost an election because he was not a member of Saddam Hussein's Ba'ath Party. The seventy-year-old man had had a hip replacement and walked with a cane. His son reported,

> They pushed him like a criminal; they didn't let him use his cane because his hands were tied. They handcuffed and put plastic hoods on my father, my uncle and my brother. I heard my father say, "I can't breathe." . . . They pushed him into the vehicle. My father was in very bad condition at that time. He couldn't talk because of the bag. . . . I could hear him gasping. . . . After that, my father stopped moving. . . . [An] officer told me my father died from a heart attack.[53]

Abed Al Razak was treated at the Abu Ghraib hospital in mid-2004, for an unspecified cardiac condition, several days before he suddenly died. Investigators carefully documented the attempted resuscitation and they noted that the body bore "no apparent signs of extraordinary trauma or injury" but they did not record whether a sandbag over his head might have impaired his breathing or prevented him from exhaling heat. It is not known whether he was subject to prolonged stress positions, Fear Up Harsh, heat or cold exposure, sleep deprivation, shouted threats, continuous loud noise, or sexual humiliation, or whether he saw a relative being beaten.[54]

Exposure to heat and cold can also cause deaths that appear to be due to natural causes. Many prisoners were forced to "stand, sit, squat, or lie down in the sand under the sun for up to three or four hours."[55] The death certificate of Tariq Mohamed Zaid attributed his death at Abu Ghraib to a "heat-related" accident without describing how he was treated prior to dying on a day when the temperature reached 130 degrees Fahrenheit.[56] An investigation was closed but has reportedly been reopened as a possible homicide by means of abusive exposure to the hot Iraqi climate and deprivation of water.[57,58] Nasef Ibrahim's death certificate says that the sixty-three-year-old, 180-pound man died of cardiovascular disease and a buildup of fluid around his heart.[59,60] However, this elderly man was stripped, doused in cold water, and kept outside in forty-degree weather for three days before becoming short of breath and suffering cardiac arrest.[61,62]

Abdureda Lafta Abdul Kareem (also known as Abu Malik Kenami) was admitted to Mosul prison on December 5, 2003, and died four days later.[63,64] Military investigators found that the short, stocky, forty-four-year-old man weighed 175 pounds. He was not medically examined before his harsh treatment. After he was interrogated, soldiers put a sandbag over his head. When he tried to remove it, the guards made him jump up and down for twenty minutes with his wrists tied in front of him, and then for twenty minutes more with his wrists bound behind his back with a plastic binder. The bound and head-bagged man was put on a mat for the night in a cell that was built for thirty prisoners but packed with sixty-six men. He was restless and "jibbering in Arabic." The guards told him to be quiet. The next morning, he was dead. Guards, medics, and two physicians noted that his eyes were very bloodshot. There were lacerations on his wrists from the plastic ties, unexplained bruises on his abdomen, and a fresh, bruised laceration on the back of his head. Army investigators noted that the body did not have defensive bruises on the arms—an odd notation, given that a man whose arms are bound behind his back cannot raise them in defense. No autopsy was performed. The death certificate lists the cause of death as "unknown." The physician at the scene surmised that Mr. Kenami died of a heart attack. It seems more likely that he suffocated because of the combined effects of how he was restrained, hooded, and positioned. Positional asphyxia looks just like death by a natural heart attack except for those telltale bloodshot eyes, which indicate conjunctival hemorrhage. Perhaps his "jibbering" was calling out for air. There are other similar cases of sudden deaths of men with little evidence of cardiac disease who were found to have unexplained facial venous congestion or pulmonary edema, also suggestive of asphyxia.[65,66]

THE DEPARTMENT OF DEFENSE RESPONDS

The Department of Defense has answered allegations of concealed homicides and needless deaths of prisoners with denials and obfuscation. It has not provided a complete list of the names, locations, and circumstances of prisoners who died by homicide, suicide, accident, or natural causes, although the Geneva Convention requires that this information be disclosed. It does not name, secure human rights monitors' visits for, or discuss the fate of persons captured by the U.S. government and turned over to other governments for imprisonment or interrogation.

In June 2004, soon after the press conference in which it released the twenty-three death certificates, Secretary of Defense Rumsfeld sent a memo reminding field commanders to comply with the existing policies for reporting and investigating prisoner deaths.[67] Two months later, in response to press reports that prisoners whom the Pentagon had claimed died of natural causes had actually died of homicides, Lieutenant Colonel Ellen Krenke cryptically asserted, "There is no evidence that *final* [emphasis added] death certificates were falsified."[68] Army Surgeon General Kevin Kiley elaborated on Krenke's statement: "An initial reported cause of death is a field expedient process, often made by local medical personnel not fully qualified to certify cause of death. Autopsies corroborate or correct initial inaccuracies."[69,70] Dr. Kiley is mistaken. Army regulations on this matter conform to civilian standards of practice: "When the cause of death is undetermined, the medical officer will make a statement to that effect. When the cause of death is finally determined, a supplemental report will be made."[71] In February 2005, the assistant secretary of defense for health affairs, Dr. William Winkenwerder, asserted that there is "no evidence" detainee death reports were falsified.[72]

Commander Craig Mallak, M.D., J.D., of the Office of the Armed Forces Medical Examiner, explained that death certificates were not promptly prepared and forwarded to an organization such as the Red Cross to distribute to families because "there was no recognized organization in Iraq with which to file death certificates nor were there families there to receive them."[73] He neglected to remind the reporters that the Geneva Convention obliges the occupying power (that is, the United States) to create such an organization.

The Defense Department rationalizes the long delay between the prompt autopsies and the final death certificates thus: "The emphasis was on getting an autopsy report out to the investigative agency, not the certificate."[74] However, the delay in finalizing death certificates enabled Pentagon officials to lie to reporters about the cause of death and thereby delay public knowledge of the homicides of prisoners. That delay violates Article 122 of the Geneva Convention:

> In all cases of occupation, each of the Parties to the conflict shall institute an official Information Bureau . . . for replying to all enquiries sent to it concerning prisoners of war, including those who have died in captivity; it will make any enquiries necessary to obtain the information which is asked for if this is not in its possession. . . . Death certificates . . . shall be forwarded as rapidly as possible to the Prisoner of War Information Bureau.

A noteworthy contrast to the U.S. delays in informing families of torture-related deaths is the case of twenty-eight-year-old Baha Mousa. British soldiers picked him up at a hotel in Basra, Iraq. A man who was imprisoned with Mr. Mousa, and later released, described what happened in prison:

> We were put in a big room with our hands tied and with bags over our heads. But I could see through some holes in my hood. Soldiers would come in—ordinary soldiers, not officers . . . [—]and they would kick us, picking on one after the other. They were kick boxing us in the chest and between the legs and in the back. We were crying and screaming. They set on Baha especially and he kept crying that he couldn't breathe in the hood. He kept asking them to take the bag off and said that he was suffocating. But they laughed at him and kicked him more. One of them said, "Stop screaming and you'll be able to breathe more easily." Baha was so scared. They increased the kicking on him and he collapsed on the floor.[75]

Three days later, Mr. Mousa's bruised body was given to his family. A British pathologist, "Professor Hill," personally told the decedent's brother that Mr. Mousa died of a beating. The British army gave the family an international death certificate listing the cause of death as "cardiorespiratory arrest: asphyxia" that has enabled the family to successfully appeal for an independent investigation.[76]

In March 2005, the report of an investigation by Vice Admiral Albert Church briefly noted his review of sixty-eight prisoner deaths from homicide and natural causes. It is impossible to cross-check the admiral's findings because he did not list the prisoners, nor did he note that his review encompassed only half of the known number of prisoners who had died.[77] Even so, Admiral Church concluded that medical personnel may have attempted to misrepresent the circumstances of the deaths of Habibullah, Dilawar, and Al-Jamadi, although he did not say how.[78]

DISCUSSION

War conspires against forensic medicine. The investigation of prisoners' deaths is not a high priority. Autopsy facilities are inadequate and often distant from prisons. Nonetheless, the Geneva Conventions' provisions requiring investigation of prisoners' deaths and public reporting of causes of death were written because of abuses that the world community, including the United States, condemned and wished to remedy. U.S. Defense Department regulations echo those conventions. Armed forces pathologists are professionally accountable under the standards of practice for investigating prisoner homicides. The "Manual on the Investigation of Torture and Other Cruel, Inhuman, or Degrading Treatment" describes that standard of medical forensic practice.[79,80] The exigencies of war do not excuse substandard postmortem exams or delays in the release of death certificates and autopsy findings while public officials misrepresent the cause and circumstances of death.

The Armed Forces Institute of Pathology bears primary responsibility for substandard investigations and reporting of prisoners' deaths. There is no evidence that its staff was trained in or followed a special protocol for evaluating prisoner deaths to ascertain whether torture took place. There is no evidence that the institute developed forms to systematically solicit information about events preceding prisoners' deaths, such as extremes of climate or whether the body was found hooded, bound, suspended, gagged, or in a stress position.

The AFIP's routine delays in completing and releasing death certificates did not comply with Army or Geneva requirements.[81] This "field expedient process," as Army Surgeon General Kiley called it, enabled Pentagon officials to falsely claim that prisoners died of natural causes after an autopsy had found homicide.[82] It invited and supported Pentagon attempts to conceal homicides and delay public knowledge of them. A medical examiner who allows a false official statement that a homicide is death by natural causes to stand for months or years is arguably an accessory after the fact if that delay obstructs the apprehension, trial, or punishment of an assailant.[83]

The medical handling of the death of Iraqi army major general Abed Hamed Mowhoush resembles the case of the Afghan taxi driver Dilawar, whose story introduced this chapter. General Mowhoush voluntarily presented himself to U.S. military authorities; he died of torture sixteen days later, on November 26, 2003.[84] Staff Sergeant Bernard Perry, commander in charge of the prison medics, and Dr. Ann Rossignol testified that on admission Major General Mowhoush received a cursory and undocumented medical interview from a medic.[85] Trial testimony tells that he was repeatedly beaten with fists, a hose, sticks, and a rifle butt under Army, Special Forces, and CIA supervision.[86] Six ribs were broken. Then, Mowhoush was stuffed headfirst into a sleeping bag that was wrapped in twenty feet of electrical wire.[87,88] A soldier crouched over Mowhoush's chest and put his hands against Mowhoush's head and then got up. A few minutes later, Mouhoush was found to have died. Sergeant Perry was summoned to the interrogation room and briefly joined other staff in attempting resuscitation.[89] Captain–Flight Surgeon Ann Rossignol was called to the interrogation room while resuscitation was in progress. She testified that she and medics Sergeant Chaheen and Captain Maria Marlow performed CPR for nearly an hour. The chief warrant officer in charge of the interrogation told Dr. Rossignol that Mowhoush was being interrogated, lost control of his urine, and collapsed; Dr. Rossignol did not ask for more details.[90] At the trial of the soldiers, she was not asked whether she saw the extensive bruising on the arms, legs, head, neck, pelvis, and front and back of the torso, or the facial blush indicative of suffocation, all of which were readily apparent to on-site investigators and to the pathologist, Dr. Michael Smith, who inspected the body.[91] A Pentagon press release cited Dr. Rossignol's opinion:

Mowhoush said he didn't feel well and subsequently lost consciousness. The soldier questioning him found no pulse, then conducted CPR and called for medical authorities. According to the on-site surgeon, it appeared Mowhoush died of natural causes.[92]

A week after the death, an autopsy found extensive trauma and concluded that General Mowhoush had died of "asphyxia due to smothering and chest compression."[93] The Office of the Armed Forces Medical Examiner withheld the death certificate until May 2004; the autopsy was made public in April 2005. This sequence of false Pentagon announcements of "natural deaths," silent acquiescence by the Office of the Armed Forces Medical Examiner, and late release of death certificates showing homicide occurred in the cases of Dilawar, Habibullah, and Al-Jamadi. It may be going on in other cases now.

Delays in finalizing death certificates have other harmful consequences. They hamper the work of those who use death certificates to question witnesses while memories are fresh. They make it impossible to comply with Geneva-mandated procedures for attempting to notify relatives of deaths so that bodies can be claimed for burial, death benefits obtained, redress sought, or closure found in learning that a loved one has died and how and when that death occurred. The Red Cross has repeatedly complained about the United States' failure to establish a system compliant with the Geneva Convention for notifying relatives of incarcerations and deaths.[94] The resulting uncertainty has compounded the suffering of thousands of Iraqi families.[95] Al-Jamadi died in November 2003, a few hours after being taken from his home as his family watched. His death certificate was finalized on May 13, 2004, as his body lay unclaimed in the Baghdad morgue.

The Office of the Armed Forces Medical Examiner failed to perform its mission to monitor deaths to identify patterns of preventable deaths.[96] Had this office promptly and publicly disclosed homicides and reported signs of abusive injuries, it would have given an authoritative early warning that something was seriously wrong in the prisons in Iraq and Afghanistan. Furthermore, in at least one instance, the office failed to preserve evidence for trial. The cooler containing autopsy specimens of a murdered prisoner, Nagen Sadoon Hatab, exploded while sitting on a hot airport tarmac awaiting transport to trial. A pathologist, Colonel Kathleen Ingwersen, then lost track of the broken hyoid (neck wishbone) showing that a soldier had grabbed and dragged Hatab by the neck and thereby strangled him. Mr. Hatab's throat and rib cage were found on two different continents. As Dr. Ingwersen explained, "I should have paid closer attention . . . instead of relying on what turned out to be a miscommunication with my assistant." She lamely suggested that she mishandled evidence because she was taking a drug to treat an allergic reaction to sandfly bites.[97] The Armed Forces Institute of Pathology then compounded the breakdown in the trial process by refusing to allow independent DNA testing to prove that the lost and found rib cage came from the decedent. The judge rebuked the institute for its lack of cooperation and the broken chain of custody.[98] Homicide charges were dropped against several defendants. One assailant was sentenced to sixty days of hard labor; another was convicted of dereliction of duty and discharged from the Marines. The mishandling of this evidence was explored as a potential challenge to the professionalism of military pathologists in the Mowhoush homicide trial.[99]

TABLE 4.1 PRISONER DEATHS BY TORTURE

Afghanistan

	NAME, AGE	DATE, LOCATION, DETAINER	EVENT HISTORY
1	???	Before September 2002, Unit ?	Army Criminal Investigative Command opened investigation on September 26, 2002, into charges of "murder," "conspiracy," and "obstruction of justice." A Commander's Report of Disciplinary or Administrative Action was administered.[100]
2	???	November 2002, salt pit, Kabul, CIA	Naked, chained, died of hypothermia, buried in unmarked, unacknowledged cemetery.[101,102] No prosecution.

NAME, AGE	DATE, LOCATION, DETAINER	EVENT HISTORY
3 Mullah Habibullah (aka Habib Ullah), ~30	Bagram, December 4, 2002, U.S. Army	Prisoner found unresponsive, restrained in his cell.[103] When a guard woke up the on-call medic to report that Habibullah had stopped breathing, medic responded, "What are you getting me for?" and told MP to call an ambulance.[104] Dr. Ingwerson did the autopsy on December 6, 2002, and promptly signed a death certificate finding homicide by "pulmonary embolism due to blunt force injury to the legs."[105] Defense Department issued false report of natural death and when pressed by media issued the death certificate in May 2004. Admiral Church identified this case as one in which medical personnel may have attempted to misrepresent the circumstances of death, possibly in an effort to disguise detainee abuse.[106] Prosecution is under way.[107,108]
4 Dilawar, 22	Bagram, December 2002, U.S. Army	See case and citations at beginning of Chapter 4, "Homicide."
5 Jamal Naseer	March 2003, Gardez, U.S. Special Forces	Severely beaten unregistered detainee. On September 20, 2004, the Army confirmed it was opening an inquiry into the death.[109]
6 Abdul Wali, 28	June 21, 2003, Asadabad, CIA	An Afghan provincial governor, who viewed the body three days after death while standing at the door of a darkened room, speculated that Mr. Wali died of a heart attack. No autopsy was performed. Former CIA contractor (civilian) and Special Operations soldier now charged with assault by beating Mr. Wali with a flashlight. Forensic investigation not released. Case referred to U.S. Department of Justice.[110,111]

NAME, AGE	DATE, LOCATION, DETAINER	EVENT HISTORY
7 Abdul Wahid	November 6, 2003, Helmand province	This person died at a U.S. prison but was arrested by Afghan militias who may have inflicted the lethal injuries before turning him over to U.S. soldiers. Dr. Kathleen Ingwersen did the autopsy and signed and finalized the death certificate on November 13, 2003. She concluded that Abdul Wahid had died by homicide from "multiple blunt force injuries complicated by probable rhabdomyolysis [extensive crush injuries of the muscles]."[112] The Pentagon released the death certificate in May 2004.
8 Sher Mohammad Khan	September 24, 2004, Khost, U.S. Army	Military officials told journalist that he had died of a heart attack within hours of being taken into custody.[113] Autopsy not released. Family retrieved the bruised body.

Iraq

NAME, AGE	DATE, LOCATION, DETAINER	EVENT HISTORY
1 Radi Nu'ma	May 8, 2003, Basra, British forces	UK soldiers delivered a note to house, "Radi Nu'ma suffered a heart attack while we were asking him questions about his son. We took him to the hospital." Family were told at the hospital that no person of that name had been admitted.[114,115] Body found in city morgue. RMP had delivered unidentified corpse on May 8 and told staff that cause of death was a heart attack but did not give any other historical or identifying information.
2 Nagen Sadoon Hatab	June 6, 2003, Camp Whitehorse, U.S. Marines	The base commander testified that a medic saw no bruises and said that Hatab was "faking" or had a "mild heart attack" when seen after a severe beating six hours before death.[116,117] The autopsy showed that Hatab had been

NAME, AGE	DATE, LOCATION, DETAINER	EVENT HISTORY
		strangled and the hyoid bone (wishbone) in his neck had been crushed.[118] (See text for details of mishandled pathologic evidence.) The coroner also found broken ribs and bruising consistent with reports of beating and kicking. Dr. Kathleen Ingwersen did the autopsy and signed and finalized the death certificate on June 10, 2003.
3 Dilar Dababa	June 13, 2003, secret center, Baghdad, U.S. Army	The circumstances of this death are not clear. Dr. Elizabeth Rouse did an autopsy on June 17, 2003, signed the death certificate characterizing the death as a homicide by "closed head injury with a cortical brain contusion and subdural hematoma."[119] However, she did not finalize the death certificate until May 14, 2004.
4 Baha Mousa (aka Baha Dawud al-Maliki)	September 13, 2003, Al Hakima, Basra, British forces	Baha Mousa was arrested and died in September 2003.[120–124] Prisoners heard him screaming. A person saw the body with lacerations, severe bruises on the chest, and a broken nose. The International Committee of the Red Cross reports that the death certificate says that death resulted from "cardio-respiratory arrest–asphyxia" of unknown cause but did not note other signs of trauma.[125] Death certificate and autopsy not available, as this death took place in British custody. British soldiers are being tried for homicide.
5 Tariq Mohamed Zaid	August 22, 2003, Iraq, U.S. Army	The sparsely documented investigation simply says that Zaid was found lying on the ground at a detention center with heatstroke. Autopsy and death certificate: "Heat related. Accidental death."[126] Dr. Michael Smith performed the autopsy and signed the death

NAME, AGE	DATE, LOCATION, DETAINER	EVENT HISTORY
		certificate on October 23, 2003, but did not finalize the death certificate until May 12, 2004. This case has now reportedly been reopened as a possible abuse by heat exposure, involving failure to provide water and shelter.[127,128]
6 Obeed Hethere Radad	September 11, 2003, Tikrit, U.S. Army	On September 10, a guard had been yelling and acting aggressively toward Mr. Radad. On September 11, Mr. Radad was in an isolation cell with his hands in flexicuffs. Mr. Radad placed his hands near concertina wire and a guard shot him in the arm and abdomen with an M-16 rifle.[129,130] The Army commander waited four days before notifying Army criminal investigators of the homicide. During this time, the base conducted a local hearing that charged a soldier with voluntary manslaughter, demoted him, and discharged him, thereby preempting the risk that he would face a more serious court-martial on the charge of unpremeditated murder.[131] Autopsy and death certificate not available.
7 Kefah [Kifah] Taha	September 17, 2003, Basra, British forces	This hotel receptionist died after three days in British custody in Basra in September.[132,133] Major James Ralph, ICU consultant at the British Military Field Hospital at Shaibah, wrote, "Admitted to our facility at 22:40 hours on 16 September. It appears he was assaulted approximately 72 hours ago and sustained severe bruising to his upper abdomen, right side of chest, left forearms and left upper inner thigh . . . acute renal failure." Death certificate and autopsy not available, as this death took place in British custody. Investigation pending.

NAME, AGE	DATE, LOCATION, DETAINER	EVENT HISTORY
8 Monadel al-Jamadi	November 4, 2003, Abu Ghraib, CIA/U.S. SEALs	Discussion and citations for this case lead Chapter 3, "Interrogation." Death certificate, based on autopsy: "Blunt force injuries complicated by compromised respiration." Dr. Jerry Hodges did the autopsy on November 9, 2003, and signed the death certificate the same day, but he did not finalize the death certificate until May 13, 2004. Admiral Church identified this case as one in which medical personnel may have attempted to conceal abuse.
9 Abed Hamed Mowhoush	November 26, 2003, FOB Tiger at Al Qaim, CIA/U.S. Army	Discussion and citations for this case in the body of Chapter 4, "Homicide." Dr. Michael Smith did an autopsy on December 2 and signed the death certificate, recording the death as a homicide by asphyxia and chest compression, on the same day. However, he did not finalize the death certificate until May 12, 2004.
10 Asad Abdul Kareem Abdul Jaleel (aka Karim Abd al-Jalil)	January 9, 2004, Fort Rifles, near Al Asad, U.S. Special Forces	Iraq army lieutenant colonel was interrogated for four days. Postmortem photographs show severe bruises. Beaten, kicked, and finally suspended with a rag in his mouth.[134] James Caruso filled out the death certificate, recording the death as a homicide from "blunt force injuries and asphyxia," on January 11, 2004, and finalized it on May 13, 2004.[135,136] The command concluded that Mr. Abd al-Jalil died from lawful force inflicted in response to repeated aggression and misconduct.

	NAME, AGE	DATE, LOCATION, DETAINER	EVENT HISTORY
11	Fashad Mohamed	April 5, 2004, Mosul, U.S. SEALs	Beaten by SEAL Team 7, interrogated and allowed to sleep and did not wake up.[137,138] Autopsy and death certificate by Dr. Elizabeth Rouse. She signed the death certificate as results "Pending" on April 26.[139] As of April 1, 2005, the cause of death remained undetermined. Multiple injuries, contusions and abrasions on body. On May 14, Dr. Rouse signed a final copy of the death certificate with no further revisions.

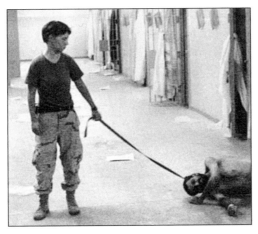

FIGURE 5.1. *Mentally ill prisoner at Abu Ghraib.*

HIS REAL NAME IS NOT KNOWN. THE MPs CALLED HIM JIHAD JERRY or Gus. He is best known as the prisoner on the leash held by MP Lynndie England in an infamous Abu Ghraib photograph that the guards posed to humiliate him.[1] Major David Ausch, M.D., the commander of Abu Ghraib's medical unit, had authorized guards to use a restraint around the abdomen for this psychotic prisoner who threw his feces and engaged in self-mutilation.[2] Dr. Ausch did not know how to use psychiatric medications and says that he could not transfer mentally ill persons to a special psychiatric facility in Iraq.[3,4] Abu Ghraib's psychiatrist worked for the BSCT (Behavior Science Consultation Team) and did not have clinical duties in the prison. Sergeant Neil Wallin, a medic, testified that Gus was often restrained and sometimes given intravenous fluids when he refused to drink.[5]

MEDICAL CARE AND PRISONERS OF WAR

Prisoners of war are at risk of neglect as much as of abuse. Many receive inadequate food, water, and medical care or live in filthy, crowded living quarters without adequate latrines, laundry, or soap and are thereby vulnerable to infectious diseases, such as dysentery, typhus, or tuberculosis. Some are inadequately sheltered from inclement weather or from shelling or sniper fire. International agreements set overlapping standards for the medical screening of incoming prisoners, for medical and dental care, for prison sanitation, food, and water, and for shelter from weapons fire. These standards are neither quaint nor are they about "fighting the last war." The United States and the Red Cross routinely cite these standards in appeals on behalf of imprisoned friends of democracy or American POWs. We back our right to invoke these rules by incorporating their provisions into our own regulations and behavior, notably "Army Regulation 190-8: Enemy Prisoners of War, Retained Personnel, Civilian Internees and Other Detainees."

In late 2003, as guards were abusing prisoners for "photo ops" at Abu Ghraib, General Ricardo Sanchez, the U.S. Army commander in Iraq, commissioned a review of Army prisons in that country. Major General Donald Ryder produced a sunny report: "Generally, conditions in prisons . . . meet minimal standards of health, sanitation, security, and human rights established by the Geneva Conventions."[6] Yet this report was sprinkled with disquieting asides. There was "no clear delineation of responsibilities for health care";[7] there was "significant variance in the health, hygiene and sanitation conditions";[8] "inadequate logistical support [was provided] for facility operations";[9] and, mental health care for Iraqi prisoners was "grossly neglected."[10] Nevertheless, General Ryder's assessment was upbeat and congratulatory: "The specifics of detainee health care, sanitation and hygiene are being addressed on a priority basis."[11] "[The] availability of medical expertise within the theater of operations . . . is exceptional."[12] "Overall, the effort at establishing a military internment . . . operation has been monumental and progressive."[13]

In mid-2004, after the Abu Ghraib photographs had been released, the acting secretary of the Army, Colonel R. L. (Les) Brownlee, directed the Army Inspector General, Lieutenant General Paul Mikolashek, to again review the prisons in Afghanistan and Iraq. The Inspector General came to a less sanguine conclusion.

> No inspected units . . . complied with all medical treatment require-
> ments . . . such as monthly height/weight screenings, chest x-rays, and
> tuberculin skin tests. . . . All interviewed medical providers stated that
> they did not have the proper equipment for treating a detainee popula-
> tion that included older chronically ill persons. . . .
>
> There was a widespread lack of preventive medicine staffing, sup-
> plies, and equipment to meet the needs of civilian prisoners and I/R [in-
> ternment/resettlement] facilities. This shortfall was compounded by
> the failure of units to deploy appropriately trained and supplied field
> sanitation teams. . . . I/R facility site selection, design and construction
> decisions did not incorporate preventive medicine considerations.
> There was significant variation in the hygiene and sanitation conditions
> throughout Afghanistan and Iraq.[14]

Lieutenant General Mikolashek found that Abu Ghraib had a

> deteriorating infrastructure that impacted the clean, safe and secure
> working environment for soldiers and living conditions for the de-
> tainees. Poor food quality and food distribution, lack of laundry capa-
> bility and inadequate personal hygiene facilities affected the detainees'
> living conditions. . . . [F]requent enemy hostile fire and lack of in depth
> force protection measures also put soldiers and detainees at risk.[15]

Health policies, outpatient records, staffing, supplies, and accountability for health and sanitation systems were seriously inadequate.[16]

Abu Ghraib's medical system was complex, understaffed, and under-equipped. The prisoners, who were incompletely segregated by category, relied on a divided medical system. The Air Force was responsible for 1,500 "military intelligence" prisoners.[17] An Army physician, an Army physician's assistant, and three to eight Army medics cared for several thousand "security detainees." In 2003, Dr. Hussain Majid, who had run Abu Ghraib's medical system under Saddam Hussein, was responsible for the common criminals.[18,19] In mid-2004, Army medic Thomas Dickson described the situation this way: "We only have like four doctors for over 8,000 detainees so you can imagine how often these guys get in to see the docs."[20] Medics treated prisoners in the cellblocks because no guards were available to escort prisoners to the clinic. Inadequately trained, or inadequately supervised, medics examined two prisoners, who unexpectedly died a few minutes after being medically cleared.[21,22] Sick diabetics were given insulin, when it was available, but the dose was not adjusted according to blood sugar.[23] As late as 2005, prisons in Iraq lacked sufficient facilities, equipment, or staff to treat prisoners with chronic diseases, disabilities, mental illness, or contagious diseases.[24] Other prisons had similar problems. In several prisons in Iraq, clinicians reused gloves, syringes, and needles, risking the spread of hepatitis or other diseases from prisoner to prisoner.[25] Human Rights Watch described a man with an untreated fracture at Kandahar in Afghanistan.[26] The Red Cross noted credible allegations of deaths from "harsh internment conditions, ill-treatment, lack of medical attention, or the combination thereof" at the Tikrit prison in Iraq.[27]

Outpatient medical records were a mess. General Mikolashek found that "none of the functions [of tracking detainees] were performed in accordance with policy. . . . There were no procedures to ensure [that] records on detainee disposition, [and] health status . . . were adequately accounted for."[28] The Army did not have training materials on maintaining medical records. Few of the prison medical staff in Iraq and Afghanistan were trained in medical recordkeeping before deployment; less than a quarter received on-the-job training.[29] In his investigation of the Abu Ghraib scandal, Major General George Fay wrote, with evident exasperation, that Abu Ghraib "medical doctors on site claim that excellent medical records were maintained. However, only a few records could be found."[30] It is reasonable to suppose that poor medical records harmed the quality of medical care, especially for chronic diseases. The next chapter will show how missing and incomplete medical records adversely affected some investigations of abuse.[31,32] In contrast to outpatient notes, hospital medical records document expert care despite shortages of surgical supplies in Iraq and Afghanistan.[33] But the prison hospitals could be difficult to get into.

Some prison physicians found that it was difficult to admit ill prisoners to hospitals for needed care. They told investigators that requests to transfer seriously ill Iraqi prisoners were administratively denied or that hospital care was given by physicians' assistants or nurse practitioners.[34] For example, a prisoner whose blood oxygen level was falling from tuberculosis in his lungs was denied hospitalization.[35] Abu Ghraib medics' notes describe prisoners with severe chest pain who were not evacuated to the hospital even though "heart attacks" were not uncommon in the hot, stressful cellblocks and prison yards.[36] It was also difficult to properly care for some prisoners who were returned to cellblocks from hospitals. After surgery, some prisoners went back to filthy cellblocks with exposed surgical pins or drains.[37–39]

TUBERCULOSIS

Tuberculosis (TB) is a pestilence of war, poverty, and prisons. It is thirty-five times more common in Iraq and seventy-two times more common in Afghanistan than in the United States.[40] It is essential to diagnose and treat tuberculosis in poor countries, where it attacks, disables, and kills people during their peak productive years. The recent emergence of drug-resistant tuberculosis has made diagnosis and treatment more important and more difficult. About 300,000 fall ill with drug-resistant tuberculosis each year. Medication for an ordinary six-month course of curative treatment for tuberculosis costs about $30; medications for drug-resistant TB cost 10 to 2,500 times as much and the disease often recurs. Many poor countries lack laboratories capable of identifying drug-resistant bacteria, clinicians who know how to use the special drugs, or the ability to pay for the expensive medicines.[41] Drug-resistant tuberculosis is especially common in prisons.[42]

Prisons are tuberculosis incubators. Close confinement and overcrowding foster TB transmission. As a result, the disease is up to a hundred times more common among prisoners than in the general population.[43,44] Tuberculosis is especially common among POWs because malnutrition, exceptionally poor health, and severe overcrowding decrease resistance to the disease. Tuberculosis spreads from prisoner to prisoner and then spreads to the population at large through discharged prisoners who acquired the disease during their confinement. Tuberculosis is so common and lethal for POWs that international law and Army regulations make it unacceptable to wait for a symptom such as coughing up blood; prisoners must be screened for tuberculosis on admission and at least annually during confinement so that infectious people can be isolated before they give the disease to their fellow internees.

The World Health Organization estimates that prewar Iraq's crumbling health system diagnosed a fifth of its citizens with contagious TB and that a small minority of these were treated. The detection and treatment rate in U.S. prisons in Iraq was worse—essentially, zero. Abu Ghraib and Camp Bucca prisons had policies for screening of newly admitted prisoners. One policy specified: "The Physician's Assistant will perform a quick exam . . . a tuberculosis test and a chest x-ray will also be given."[45] Those screening policies were not implemented.

Hussain Mohammed Basim was not screened for tuberculosis when he was imprisoned at Camp Cropper, near the Baghdad airport.[46,47] In July 2003, he coughed up blood and was taken to the infirmary, where tuberculosis was diagnosed and treatment started. The highly infectious prisoner was sent back to the crowded prison compound, where he died the next day of massive tubercular bleeding into his lungs. The record of the subsequent investigation does not show that the military medics who attempted to resuscitate him in the prison yard knew of his diagnosis. The investigators do not describe any effort to screen prisoners, medics, guards, or interrogators who were exposed to Mr. Basim for TB, as required by standard medical practice and Army regulations.[48] Basim's case is exceptional, in that even though Camp Cropper did not screen for tuberculosis, a physician had stockpiled some antituberculosis drugs after a child had died of tubercular bleeding into his lungs. That child's death was never reported; it is noted in passing in an obscure footnote.[49]

Two months after Mr. Basim died, General Geoffrey Miller complained about the prisons in Iraq, "Some detainees who had infectious medical conditions were detained in the general internee population. This mingling of internees could result in possible contamination of other detainees and soldier detention staff." He recommended establishing "special needs sections" for "internees with contagious medical conditions."[50] Three months later, in December 2003, Camp Bucca in Iraq still did not have any means of diagnosing TB. In mid-2004, the Army Inspector General found that none of thirty-six prisons in Iraq or Afghanistan even performed chest X rays to screen for tuberculosis.[51] Given this claim, it is hard to explain an FBI, State Department, and military health assessment that found a comprehensive tuberculosis program operating at the Shiberghan prison in Afghanistan in April 2003.[52] Prison pharmacies in Iraq and Afghanistan were not stocked with drugs for treating tuberculosis.[53]

MENTAL HEALTH

Medical and military personnel, FBI agents, and Red Cross observers observed many prisoners at Guantánamo Bay, in Iraq, and in Afghanistan suffering from severe mental illness.[54–58] Some had preexisting mental conditions. Others became ill from overcrowding, fear, mistreatment, and the stress of indefinitely long imprisonment. Red Cross medical experts saw prisoners suffering from stress-induced impairments in concentration, memory, and speech, as well as anxiety and suicidal inclinations. For example, a Red Cross team described a severely mentally ill prisoner in an Abu Ghraib isolation cell whose pulse was 120 beats per minute and who did not respond to verbal or painful stimuli.[59]

Major General Ryder's 2003 investigation of U.S. prisons in Iraq noted, "The mentally ill were receiving no treatment. . . . Mental illness is a grossly neglected area for the health care of Iraqi detainees."[60] Prison pharmacies rarely stocked medications for major psychiatric conditions.[61]

Medics and nurses, not physicians, treated prisoners who were so ill as to merit hospitalization.[62] General Miller complained of Abu Ghraib: "Detainees suffering from apparent mental illness were segregated in a holding pen that was normally used for disciplinary purposes." He suggested developing "special needs sections"[63] for mentally ill prisoners, as he had for those with TB. Nothing happened. Medical records show little treatment of severe mental illness. A typical clinic note from Mosul, Iraq, states,

> 34-year-old Iraqi prisoner brought from detention center for evaluation of bizarre behavior. MP medics report detainee refusing medications. Soiling self with urine. Also, MPs express concern regarding skin lesions . . . patient will not cooperate with examination but does not resist efforts to examine him. Instructions: 1) discontinue [anticonvulsant], 2) start [another anticonvulsant], 3) Begin olanzepine [an antipsychotic], 4) Return if detainee develops arm lesions.[64]

That patient should have had a medical plan for evaluating the response of the psychotic symptoms to the medication. There should have been an assessment of whether the prisoner had a condition like schizophrenia or had broken down in the prison. Instead, the follow-up plan focused on "arm lesions."

Severely mentally ill prisoners were treated in degrading ways at Guantánamo and in prisons in Iraq. Abu Ghraib guards took still and video photographs of prisoners who smeared themselves with feces, consumed or threw feces or urine, or inserted objects, for example, a banana, in their rectums.[65] Sergeant Neil Wallin, a medic, discussed a videotape of an Abu Ghraib prisoner known as Shitboy. The tape shows the prisoner repeatedly slamming his head against the wall.[66] Lieutenant Colonel Steven Jordan, who was responsible for the Interrogation and Debriefing Center at Abu Ghraib, says that a Dr. Anderson, a military physician, knew that this man was in the cellblock and needed psychiatric care.[67] He also says that he and Dr. Anderson asked Colonel Jerry Phillabaum, commander of Abu Ghraib's military police, to move "mentally unstable" prisoners out of the cellblock, to no avail.[68] Some guards would compel inmates who smeared feces on themselves to roll in the dirt before hosing them off with cold water.[69] At Camp Bucca in Iraq, the Army Surgeon General confirmed a report that psychotic prisoners were lying in their feces and urine in metal storage containers where the air temperature reached 130 degrees.[70] Regressed inmates were beaten at Guantánamo for being uncooperative.[71] MPs at Bagram, in Afghanistan, nicknamed a mentally ill prisoner who ate his feces and cut himself with concertina wire "Timmy," after a disabled child in the animated television show *South Park*. They kicked and suspended him and made him cry out in a voice that mimicked his "namesake."[72]

The Defense Department concealed many suicide attempts under the opaque jargon "manipulative self injurious behavior." This included most of 120 "hanging gestures" at Guantánamo, one of which caused "severe brain damage."[73,74] In January 2004, the government classified only two of twenty-three self-hangings as attempted suicides.[75] Military physicians silently acquiesced in this unusual misdiagnostic term. Overall, the government claims that there have been only thirty-six suicide attempts by twenty-two Guantánamo prisoners.[76] Abd al-Rahman attempted suicide at Camp Bucca in Iraq after months of torture, despairing of his release.[77] Suicidal behavior, like other symptoms of mental illness, could result in harsher treatment. Muhammad Naim Farooq told Amnesty International of seeing two men kept nude in solitary confinement after unsuccessfully attempting to hang themselves with their clothing at Guantánamo. The Defense Department did not answer Amnesty International's February 2003 request that it evaluate whether prison conditions were contributing to the many suicide attempts.[78]

FOOD

Malnutrition is a regular feature of prisoner-of-war camps. American soldiers starved in Japanese prisons during World War II. Serbs starved prisoners in the recent war in the former Yugoslavia. International law and Army Regulations require prison authorities to provide adequate food and to weigh inmates monthly to confirm that they are not becoming malnourished by underfeeding or through inability to get a fair portion of the distributed food. Medical professionals are responsible for monitoring the adequacy of prison feeding.

The meal system at Abu Ghraib was in chaos.[79,80] Corrupt private contractors failed to deliver the contracted amount of food. Prison commanders did not have the authority to issue or enforce the food supplier contracts. Outside commanders ignored information about the breakdown. Major David Dinenna, of Abu Ghraib's Military Police Battalion, engaged in this e-mail exchange with a senior military police commander:[81]

October 27, 2003, 9:50 AM: Major [William] Green . . . While I am addressing basic necessities; Contract Meals. Disaster. . . . Short hundred of meals every feeding, bugs and dirt are found in the meals several times a week and for the past two days prisoners have been vomiting after they eat. That coupled with the fact that their arrival time varies tremendously. This is of great concern as Ramadan [when meals may only be eaten after sunset] has begun. We are now out of [field rations] for the prisoners.

October 27, 11:09 AM. Major Green to Major Dinenna: The contractor has people with the food from the kitchen to your site. They eat the meals and I would like to know who from your staff is inspecting the food before it goes to the prisoners? Who is making the charges that there is dirt, bugs or whatever in the food? If it is the prisoners, I would take that with a grain of salt.

October 27, 11:20 AM. Major Dinenna to Major Green: Food is not just late, there isn't enough. Our MPS, medics and field surgeon can easily identify, bugs, krats [sic; other context suggests the reference is to rodent feces or cockroaches] and dirt and they did.

Nov 2, 7:48 AM. Major Dinenna writes: ALCON [All Concerned], Have you ever experienced about 80 prisoners standing in line at 2130 hours at night, cold and being told the venders do not have any more food? Well this is becoming a nightly routine. . . . Why is it so difficult to bring enough food? That is what the MPs are asking every meal due to the fact that they, not you, or me, have to deal with it every day. So I guess my question is, who in the hell can fix this so that we can at least give the soldier the basic necessary tools to guard prisoners, without having to worry about a riot, fight, or other related problems in the compounds during meal time?

At Kandahar in Afghanistan, food sanitation was also "extremely poor."[82]

Command Sergeant Major Joseph Arrison, also of an Abu Ghraib MP battalion, testified what happened when prisoners were given Army field rations because of the shortage of prison food. "I saw where, because of the Iraqi's strict forbiddance of pork products, they were throwing away the military field rations because they included jambalaya and pork chops."[83] The Army maintains that the distribution of pork to Muslims was an emergency measure; however, it seems to fit into a broad pattern of disrupting prayer rituals with interrogations and mishandling the Koran. The U.S. Army Muslim chaplain James Yee was regularly and inexcusably given pork meals while imprisoned in the United States on a false charge of treason.[84]

There was little oversight of the adequacy of food rations. At Camp Bucca, food was distributed, long after having been prepared, from thirty-gallon drums. Prisoners served themselves by dipping personal containers of various sizes into the communal pots.[85] There was no oversight of food distribution to ensure that each prisoner was receiving sufficient food to prevent malnutrition. Few prisons in Iraq or Afghanistan conducted the Geneva Convention's mandated monthly weighing of prisoners to ensure that stigmatized or weak prisoners did not become malnourished.

HUNGER STRIKES

Prisoner hunger strikes pose a difficult problem for prison health personnel. Most hunger strikes are individual affairs. A particular prisoner, usually of some prominence so that he or she can draw public attention, refuses food to seek some kind of relief such as the right to see relatives, communicate, make a public statement, or not be mistreated.[86–88] Prison hunger strikes are a form of political expression; refusal of food is often the only form of expression available to a prisoner. Few hunger strikers are suicidal although a substantial minority will fast to death or succumb from the lingering effects of a fast.[89] British prisoners from Northern Ireland and, more recently, general prisoners in Turkey have staged collective hunger strikes in which a group of prisoners stops eating. Sometimes, the prisoners commence their fast together; sometimes they stop eating in staggered relays so that new groups of critically ill prisoners emerge over a more extended time. Collective hunger strikes are coordinated by prisoners' committees. Compared to individual strikes, they raise a new issue: is the individual participant, however rational, a volunteer, or has he or she been coerced into joining the strike by other prisoners?

To further complicate matters, few hunger strikers refuse all food and water, a drastic action that would quickly lead to death. Most hunger strikers take fluids plus insufficient amounts of food, with the aim of allowing public pressure to build and dialogue to occur, so that a compromise can resolve the dispute behind the strike. This slow starvation creates a new medical problem. Chronic malnutrition can lead to irreversible nerve, brain, and heart damage even if the strike is terminated. Strikers need medical information about what vitamins to take in order to increase their chance of recovering from a terminated strike without severe permanent disability.

Prison clinicians are caught between the prisoners' rights and prison officials' priorities. Officials see strikes as a security disturbance, a threat to the health of the prisoners, and something to address forcefully, by placing feeding tubes into the stomachs of restrained prisoners if necessary.[90–92] Some courts have supported this view. Physicians value the saving of life, although medical ethics strongly counsels against forcing treatment on competent persons who do not want it. Furthermore, if a hunger strike is motivated by the desire to stop torture, forced feeding is abusive mistreatment, essentially a way to revive the prisoner for continued abuse.[93] The tension between the wishes of the prisoner-patients and the prison officials ensured that hunger strikes in Iraq and Guantánamo would severely test medical ethics. The 1975 World Medical Association's Declaration of Tokyo proposes the most respected view of medical ethics on this matter.

Where a prisoner refuses nourishment and is considered by the doctor as capable of forming an unimpaired and rational judgment concerning the consequences of such voluntary refusal of nourishment, he or she shall not be fed artificially. The decision as to the capacity of the prisoner to form such a judgment should be confirmed by at least one other independent doctor. The consequences of the refusal of nourishment shall be explained by the doctor to the prisoner.

The World Medical Association's 1991 Declaration of Malta details the responsibilities of physicians who are faced with a hunger-striking prisoner. Physicians must assess whether the prisoner is making a rational decision. This includes assessing whether the decision is voluntary and not coerced. A trusting and confidential relationship between the prisoner and the physician is necessary if the physician is to assess coercion by other prisoners. Prison officials tend to regard medical confidentiality that protects information as to the coordination of a hunger strike as conflicting with prison security. The doctor must then inform the prisoner of the consequences of a hunger strike, such as permanent nerve damage. In this context, the ethics of informed consent oblige the physician to tell the prisoner-patient about vitamins that can reduce the risk of this damage. Again, prison officials are reluctant to accept the principle that a physician should advise a prisoner on how to conduct a strike with minimal risk of brain, nerve, and heart damage.[94]

Government documents show isolated accounts of individual hunger strikes in Iraq in 2003 and 2004. The motivation behind these actions is unclear. Some may simply have been engendered by the quality or kind of food. In mid-August 2003, Dham Spah died after an eight-day "hunger strike," because he would not eat American food.[95,96] Five days earlier, Mohammed Najem Abed, about sixty years old, also died at Abu Ghraib after a two-day hunger strike. He reportedly suffered chest pains and collapsed in the prison yard; an autopsy concluded that he died of heart disease complicated by diabetes. The twenty-page report of the forensic investigation details Abed's cardiac arrest but gives no information on his hunger strike.[97,98] Forced intravenous fluids were given in isolated instances, such as the mentally ill Gus mentioned at the beginning of this chapter.[99] A medic at Bagram told how he administered intravenous fluids to prisoners who "refused to drink water as a result of a cultural belief."[100] Intravenous solutions hydrate but they do not nourish. Army investigators did not ask or note whether the medics added vitamins to intravenous fluids in order to prevent nerve and brain damage.

A series of collective hunger strikes erupted with a fury at Guantánamo in mid-2005 and continue in early 2006, as this book nears publication.[101] Up to a quarter or third of the prisoners, 130 hunger strikers, have participated.[102] About 20 percent of these are tube fed. The Defense Department has not allowed the hunger strikers to speak to the press or medical observers about their motivations. Sufficient time has not elapsed to allow the official records describing these strikes to be declassified. Accordingly, most information comes from lawyers and human rights groups although Pentagon spokespersons have confirmed aspects of media accounts concerning force feeding and approximate number of participants in the strikes. The principal grievances are prison abuses and indeterminate confinement. A former Guantánamo prisoner, Suleiman Shah, explained it this way: "All of the people were worried about how long we would be there for. People were becoming mad because they were saying: 'When will they release us? They should take us to the high court.'" Many, including Suleiman, stopped eating.[103]

The Defense Department enlisted its medical staff in a program of force feeding. Echoing the views of the assistant secretary of defense for health affairs, Dr. William Winkenwerder, Jr., and of the base commander, the military physician Captain John Edmondson asserted, "I will not allow them to do harm to themselves."[104] Dr. Edmondson says that the military physicians are "screened" before deployment to Guantánamo "to ensure that they do not have ethical objections to force feedings." The clinicians assessed the nutritional status of striking prisoners and decided when involuntary feeding should be undertaken. Clinicians inserted feeding tubes through the nose, down the esophagus, and into the stomach. If X rays were required to confirm that the feeding tube was in the stomach rather than in the lungs, radiographers were also part of the system of forced feeding. The clinicians monitored the feedings to normalize nutritional laboratory parameters while their patients' arms, shoulders, legs, and waists were strapped to a chair whose manufacturer advertises it as a "padded cell on wheels."[105]

SANITATION

The Mosul Collection Center in Iraq was designed to hold two or three prisoners. It would have been easy to meet sanitation standards there if the Army had not put as many twenty-seven prisoners in its two small pens.[106] Each pen had a six-by-twelve-foot roof to provide shelter from the Iraqi sun and one exposed plastic tank that served as a toilet. The prisoners were not given enough water to wash themselves or their clothes. Some wore the same clothes for more than two months. A Pentagon e-mail explained the failed sanitation at forward bases like Mosul this way: "Lower echelon units [are] capturing and detaining individuals for long periods of time (in violation of doctrine, but critical to obtain timely intel [intelligence] in a HUMINT-driven [human intelligence] operation), support elements are inadequately structured to maintain the infrastructure."[107]

In 2004, in the wake of the release of the Abu Ghraib photographs, the Army described the sanitation systems in its prisons in Iraq and Afghanistan in dire terms. The report cited

[a] lack of preventive medicine staffing, supplies and equipment. . . . Medical leaders responsible for direct oversight of preventive medicine personnel lacked specific training in detainee operations and field sanitation. . . . There were no theater or unit level policies that addressed preventive medicine requirements for detainee operations. . . . [There] was no evidence of specific medical planning for field sanitation/preventive medicine support to detainee operations.[108]

All but one of thirty-six prisons lacked the "properly trained and equipped field sanitation teams" that Army regulations required.[109–111]

Many prisons were sties. Abu Ghraib's tent compounds were erected over an old landfill and garbage migrated up through the soil. Rats and feral dogs roamed its living areas. There was standing water around the latrines and in the tent compound.[112,113] In one compound, seven hundred prisoners ran through twelve showers in two hours.[114] At Bucca prison, water spigots were a few feet from exposed sewage.[115] At Bagram, hand-carried latrine buckets spilled human waste onto the floor.[116] The Army characterized prison water systems throughout Iraq as having

> poor lines, poor pressure, line breaks, and cross connections and back flow.... Same scenario for sewer systems. Jail cells with open sewer "trenches" backed up sewer lines in cells, etc add to the rodent populations, ants, roaches, etc.... With no place to eat, drink, shower, etc other than in their cells, how do we keep proper sanitation alive? The jails have no other rooms to use, barely space as it is for them to sleep. This causes even more problems as you can imagine.[117]

Poor sanitation was a precipitant for riots that were suppressed with lethal force.[118,119] In June 2004, Abu Ghraib prisoners complained of long and indeterminate internments, inadequate housing, and the lack of showers, shampoo, blankets, and toilets. Some prisoners threw stones at guards on the observation towers. First Sergeant Daryl Keithley and Captain Troy Armstrong told the prisoners that their questions would be answered when information became available. The next afternoon, thirty to forty detainees demonstrated again; some threw stones. MPs responded with 12-gauge shotguns and M-16s, killing one prisoner and wounding seven others. Army investigators concluded that the guards acted properly in response to a credible threat of serious injury or death. They recommended more barbed wire and patrols, removal of rocks from the prison grounds, and the posting of rules in Arabic and English. The investigators also suggested "proper life support for prisoners (hygiene support and supplies)," but nothing was done about these issues.[120]

EXPOSURE TO ORDNANCE

Prisoners are not to be exposed to bombardment, snipers, or other military hazards. The Geneva Convention Relative to the Protection of Civilian Persons in Time of War, which was supposed to govern prisons in Iraq,

puts it this way: "The Detaining Power shall not set up places of internment in areas particularly exposed to the dangers of war." U.S. Army Regulation 190-8 on POW camps has a similar requirement.

Brigadier General Janis Karpinski, the commander of the military police at Abu Ghraib from 2003 until 2004, warned Major General Geoffrey
Miller when he selected Abu Ghraib in 2003 to be a major interrogation
center that the prison was attacked three or four times each week.[121,122]
Colonel Thomas Pappas, the senior Army Intelligence officer, also knew
that Abu Ghraib was frequently attacked.[123] General Ricardo Sanchez's
office recieved numerous updates on mortar, rocket-propelled grenade,
and small arms fire on the prison.[124] General Karpinski openly complained to the press about the danger after Abu Ghraib was made into an
interrogation center.[125] General Karpinski and the Red Cross regularly
complained about the mortar, grenade, and small arms fire raining down
on Abu Ghraib prisoners who lived in unprotected tents encircled by concertina wire.[126-128] A safer and logistically well-supported alternative
prison existed at Camp Bucca in south Iraq.[129] There is no evidence that
the Defense Department ever considered moving the Abu Ghraib prisoners to a safer location. The threat to the prisoners was ignored.

The Army did take steps to protect the Abu Ghraib guards. Maps
showed the areas where mortar and sniper attacks were most common.[130]
An MP orientation program slide contained the following advice:

> IED [improvised explosive device] and RPG [rocket-propelled grenade]
> threats in the area are high. . . . Mortar threat is high toward Abu G.
> Bring your flak vest and Kevlar with you every morning, you never know
> how long your day will last. Don't be without your gear when the mor-
> tars fall, even your best friend will become reluctant to share.[131]

A year later, the Army Inspector General's investigation of the Abu
Ghraib scandal concluded, "Abu Ghraib was determined to be undesir-
able for housing detainees because it is . . . under frequent hostile fire,
placing soldiers and detainees at risk. . . . Abu Ghraib's location goes
against doctrine for setting up Internment/Resettlement facilities."[132]

The number of prisoner casualties from mortars, rocket-propelled grenades, and sniper fire has not been disclosed. Six died in one attack in 2003; at least twenty-two died in an attack in 2004.[133,134] Hundreds have been wounded. Abu Ghraib was heavily shelled in April 2005. The Defense Department has not released a casualty account for those attacks, but *Stars and Stripes* quoted a nurse as saying that there were between 110 and 120 casualties.[135]

THE DEPARTMENT OF DEFENSE RESPONDS

In 2005, senior Pentagon health officials, including Army Surgeon General Kiley, asserted, "Medical personnel examine prisoners upon their incarcerations and clear them as fit for confinement. If a prisoner is found not to be fit . . . the prisoner receives appropriate medical treatment in accordance with the standards of care for all patients—including those for military personnel."[136] Ironically, Dr. Kiley's statement came as his office issued a report that essentially confirmed the dismal findings of the Army Inspector General's 2004 assessment. The Surgeon General's report claimed that substantial improvements had been made over the preceding year.[137] David Tornberg, M.D., M.P.H., the deputy assistant secretary of defense for health affairs, took a harder position. He denied that military intelligence clinicians have a physician-patient relationship and asserted that they have no obligation to treat anything except "life-threatening emergencies."[138]

DISCUSSION

The Defense Department failed to meet prisoners' health needs. Prison medical and health systems in Iraq and Afghanistan were understaffed and underequipped. There was no screening for tuberculosis; undiagnosed and untreated cases needlessly endangered prisoners, soldiers, and the broader community. Water was inadequate for personal hygiene. Food was filthy; supervision of portion sizes and weight loss was poor. There was virtually no planning to address the predictable need for a prison health and sanitation infrastructure. Demoralization from neglected basic needs contributed to riots and hunger strikes that were suppressed with force. Many medical officers were unaware of Army prison health regulations. Defense Department policies were vague, mutually contradictory, or nonexistent.[139] No health policy for Iraq or Afghanistan was written until 2004, two years after the invasion of Afghanistan and a year after that of Iraq.[140]

The treatment of mental illness was worse than inadequate. The prisons were designed to be psychiatrically destructive.[141] General Miller's policy of using guards to "set the conditions" for interrogation was designed to create sleep-deprived, stressed, degraded, and isolated prisoners. Interrogation plans for Fear Up and Ego Down were designed to engender anxiety, fear, and hopelessness. Poor sanitation, overcrowding, indeterminate detention, and, in some cases, shelling and sniper fire aggravated prisoners' distress. Prisoners became demoralized, depressed, regressed and withdrawn, psychotic and suicidal. As the United Nations Working Group assessed Guantánamo,

> These conditions have led in some instances to serious mental illness, over 350 acts of self-harm in 2003 alone, individual and mass suicide attempts and widespread, prolonged hunger strikes. The severe mental health consequences are likely to be long term in many cases, creating health burdens on detainees and their families for years to come.[142]

The Defense Department's February 2005 claim that "psychological care also is available for [Guantánamo] detainees who need it or request it" is profoundly misleading.[143] As a Guantánamo interpreter, Sergeant Erik Saar, succinctly put it, "It was a little ridiculous that the psych team was trying to conduct damage control for everything the interrogators were trying to do and I found that . . . there were certain detainees the psych techs didn't see because the interrogators wanted those guys depressed and dejected."[144]

Prisoners of war are inherently in a precarious position. Military priorities take precedence over stigmatized enemies for access to limited resources. Nevertheless, the history of the abusive neglect of prisoners of war was the impetus for international law and Defense Department standards for POW camps. It would be unfair to condemn the Defense Department for isolated deficiencies; it would be wrong to excuse systematic failures by hailing proper treatment in a few showcase locations. Sixty to ninety percent of the prisoners in Iraq and a similar proportion in Guantánamo were of no intelligence value or had committed no crime.[145,146] The exigencies of war do not exempt the Defense Department from accountability to the basic needs of innocent, ignorant, and guilty prisoners. The department is properly judged.

The response of military clinicians to these problems must be looked at with a discriminating eye. The investigations do show clinicians complaining about insufficiency of staff and medical supplies and about the difficulty of getting prisoners admitted to the field hospitals. Some physicians, like the one who set up a stockpile of antituberculosis drugs after a child died of the disease, secured supplies outside regular inventories.[147] Another stopped notifying the Abu Ghraib hospital of impending transfers of prisoners because of the hospital's refusal to preapprove admissions.[148] There were occasional medical protests with regard to psychiatric care and feeding.

The declassified documents do not show clinicians advocating for prisoners whose health was endangered by poor sanitation or exposure to mortar and sniper fire. However, such complaints about the inadequately supplied medical system must be distinguished from their silence as to the medical implications of human rights systematic failures in health care, sanitation, psychiatric care, tuberculosis screening and treatment, feeding, and protection from armament fire.

The responsibility for prisoners' health and the healthfulness of their living conditions falls squarely on medical personnel. The UN's "Principles of Medical Ethics Relevant to the Role of Health Personnel, Particularly Physicians, in the Protection of Prisoners and Detainees Against Torture and Other Cruel, Inhuman or Degrading Treatment or Punishment" describes the fundamental obligations of prison clinicians this way.

> Principle 1: Health personnel, particularly physicians, charged with the medical care of prisoners and detainees, have a duty to provide them with protection of their physical and mental health and treatment of disease. . . .

Principle 6: There may be no derogation from the foregoing principles on any ground whatsoever, including public emergency.

The UN Standard Minimum Rules for the Treatment of Prisoners define
prison medical officers' responsibility this way:

> The medical officer shall report to the director whenever he considers
> that a prisoner's physical or mental health has been or will be injuri-
> ously affected by continued imprisonment or by any condition of im-
> prisonment. The medical officer shall regularly inspect and advise the
> director upon: (a) The quantity, quality, preparation and service of food;
> (b) The hygiene and cleanliness of the institution and the prisoners; (c)
> The sanitation . . . of the institution . . .

The UN "Declaration on the Protection of All Persons from Being Subjected to Torture and Other Cruel, Inhuman or Degrading Treatment or
Punishment" says that "pain or suffering . . . from prison conditions that
do not comply with the Standard Minimum Rules may, in some circumstances, constitute torture."

Where does medical responsibility for this violation of human rights
lie? Vice Admiral Church blamed field personnel for poor health and
sanitation systems, although he conceded that "few U.S. personnel . . . had
received specific training relevant to detainee screening and medical
treatment."[149] He did not mention the Defense Department's underlying
failure to provide adequate medical or sanitation matériel, staff, or staff
training, or to ensure that health systems were held accountable to Army
regulations and Geneva requirements. A historical precedent may be
helpful.

The conditions at Defense Department prisons in Iraq and Afghanistan
uncomfortably echo the scandal about prisons during the U.S. Civil War.
The Union and the Confederacy both operated overcrowded POW
camps that failed to provide proper sanitation, medical care, food, and
shelter. An estimated 50,000 to 60,000 persons may have died at Alton,
Andersonville, Camp Douglas, Point Lookout, Belle Isle, Salisbury, Rock
Island, Camp Chase, and other prisons across the Union and Confeder-

ate states. Although these deaths vastly outnumber those in the Defense Department's current prisons in Iraq and Afghanistan, medical care, sanitation, food storage, overall human longevity, and military logistics have also greatly improved over the last 140 years. The rationales invoked to explain and justify the Civil War prisons' conditions resemble those that appear in government records today. War departments feared that released prisoners would return to combat. Various parties fairly and unfairly blamed logistical barriers, corrupt provisioners, genocidal neglect, and the commandants of the deficient camps. Like Major Dinenna, who appealed for food for Abu Ghraib, Major Eugene Sanger, the surgeon in charge of Elmira, unsuccessfully petitioned the Union War Department for more supplies. Captain Henry Wirz, a physician's assistant who was the commander of Andersonville, asked an unresponsive Confederacy for better shelter, food, and medical supplies. He was hanged after the war for conspiring to "impair and injure the health and destroy the lives of large numbers of Federal prisoners." Today, senior officers, such as Admiral Church, blame local officers like Major David Dinenna, as their predecessors blamed Dr. Sanger or Captain Wirz. One hundred and fifty years later, the Civil War POW camps still evoke shame and anger.

Command responsibility for the prison health systems lies with the assistant secretary of defense for health affairs, William Winkenwerder, M.D.; with Dr. Winkenwerder's deputy assistant secretary, David Tornberg, M.D., M.P.H.; and with the Army Surgeon General, Kevin Kiley, M.D. The 2004 Army Inspector General's report directed its reform suggestions to MEDCOM, the Army Medical Command, which is immediately responsible for sanitation, food, water, and medical services for the prisons in Iraq and Afghanistan.[150] The inspector general did not, however, investigate or name the MEDCOM unit or its senior officer. That responsibility lies with the 3rd MEDCOM, based in Decatur, Georgia, about 125 miles from the site of the prison camp at Andersonville. Three months after the Army Inspector General's report, President Bush promoted 3rd MEDCOM's commander, Army brigadier general Ronald Silverman, to the rank of major general.

CHAPTER 6

SILENCE

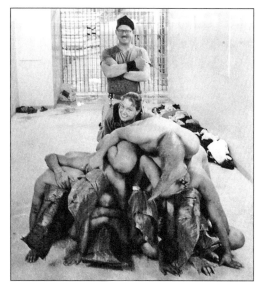

FIGURE 6.1. *Pyramid of prisoners at Abu Ghraib.*

SHORTLY AFTER MIDNIGHT ON NOVEMBER 7, 2003, A GROUP OF ABU Ghraib guards put sandbags on seven prisoners' heads, ordered them to strip, and forced them into a "dog pile."[1,2] Over the next twenty minutes, one or two soldiers jumped on the pile a couple of times and stomped on the prisoners' fingers and toes and feet.[3-6] They also passed around cameras and took turns posing by the pyramid. Some of the photographs were posted, with other pictures of abuse, on computers where many other soldiers saw them.[7-12] One prisoner, a man who had been arrested for car theft, felt someone place a foot on his head. "He put his whole weight on my head and on my knee. I was screaming and crying. . . . I wanted to kill myself. . . . I felt humiliated but I had nothing to kill myself with."[13] Sergeant Ivan "Chip" Frederick testified, "I didn't think anyone cared about what happened to the detainees as long as they did not die."[14] Guard Jeremy Sivits, who became the first Abu Ghraib guard to be court-martialed for abusing prisoners, recalled, "We would joke around, everyone would laugh at the things we had them do."[15]

Guard Charles Graner cradled a prisoner's head in his arm and struck him on the head.[16] The prisoner fell to the ground. "Damn, that hurt," said Graner.[17,18] Then, Sergeant Frederick drew an X with his finger on another prisoner's chest and struck him hard.[19-21] The prisoner pointed to his chest, fell to his knees breathing heavily and collapsed to the floor. The guards were afraid that he was dying and summoned a medic.[22,23] Nurse Helga Margot Aldape-Moreno came to the cellblock. She testified that she saw a "pyramid of naked guys who had sandbags over their heads . . . almost like cheerleaders," and that she heard guards yelling at them.[24-26] She examined the collapsed man, who, she told investigators, had had an "anxiety attack," and left him in the room with the others.[27] She did not evacuate the prisoner for medical care or report the beating or the pyramid of naked, crying prisoners. In 2004, Army investigators suggested that she be disciplined for failing to report the abuse.[28] In 2005, in response to public descriptions of this case and despite the sworn statements, testimony, and investigations, the Army Surgeon General claimed that his "team found no evidence to verify or disprove this allegation about the nurse's passive acquiescence to the abuse she saw."[29]

A simple question led to this book: where were the doctors and nurses at Abu Ghraib? Why didn't medical personnel blow the whistle on the abuse and neglect of prisoners that had been taking place long before the Abu Ghraib scandal became public? This chapter tries to describe the silence of medical command leaders, deployed clinicians, and medical societies in the United States.

Silence about abuse has two general forms: failing to see abuse for what it is, and failing to act when abuse is seen. For an investigator, silence is like dark matter, difficult to detect and harder to measure. The silent parties do not acknowledge or document their silence. A witness may report that an abusive soldier and a doctor agreed not to record the fact or cause of a prisoner's injury, but such anecdotes do not reveal whether the arrangements were routine or exceptional. Still, it is possible to infer a deep silence from the duration and extent of the known abuses. An Army psychiatrist, Dr. Henry Nelson, assessed Abu Ghraib this way: "The worst human qualities and behaviors came to the fore and a pervasive dominance came to prevail. . . . The sadistic and psychopathic behavior was appalling and shocking. . . . The Military Intelligence unit seemed to be operating in a conspiracy of silence."[30]

Investigations describe clinicians who could not "see" abuse. A Navy medic, Petty Officer Blay, watched a guard slap and punch numerous prisoners at Camp Whitehorse in Iraq. Petty Officer Blay said that the beatings, which made the men groan and stagger, were meant to get the prisoners "to know that these people were now in charge." He did not report the beatings because he felt that they were reasonable.[31] Another medic, Sergeant Wallin, also did not report seeing detainees being slapped, hit, or forced to go nude or to wear women's underwear on their heads.[32]

The records also show instances of clinicians who failed to rise to the responsibility of confronting abusive acts. A Navy medic "walked away" when he saw soldiers abusing prisoners.[33] Medic Reuben Layton saw pictures of nude male and female detainees posted on a personal computer at Abu Ghraib, but he did not report them because military intelligence people were in the pictures.[34] In another case, he went partway, asking guards to stop beating Al-Sheikh's wounded leg and to not suspend him from his injured shoulder, but he did not report the abuse, when he saw it repeated on two more occasions.[35] In late 2003, the medic Sergeant Wallin was called to a cell after Abu Ghraib guards slammed a prisoner known as one of the "Three Stooges" into a wall, lacerating his chin. He saw the prisoner with a sandbag over his head and blood running down his clothes from a two-and-a-half-inch cut. He saw "blood on the wall near a metal weld, which I believed to be the place where the detainee received his injury." He sutured the wound with thirteen stitches but did not report it because he said that he did "not know how he was injured or if it was done by himself or another."[36] Major Anthony Cavallaro of the military police summarized this kind of moral passivity thus: "What bothered me most about what happened at Abu Ghraib was that no soldier came forward and said this is wrong."[37]

Physicians are responsible for collecting medical evidence from injured patients who report being assaulted. Investigations are compromised if that opportunity is missed. Bruises disappear; fractures heal; memories dim; witnesses move on. A physician's job includes describing and, if possible, photographing injuries. The physician should write down the patient's description of the assailant and his or her account of how and when the injuries were inflicted. An Abu Ghraib record that did meet that standard recorded a prisoner's story of beatings, stress positions, being forced underwater until he vomited, and being sodomized with an "industrial penis." It recorded the prisoner's description of the assailants. The physician correlated that patient's story with the findings on the medical examination and that record served as evidence in an investigation.[38]

Such records were the exception, not the rule. Red Cross medical monitors described a number of prisoners with injuries from beatings or burns that had not been recorded in clinical notes.[39] In 2003, American soldiers arrested Sadiq Zoman and imprisoned him at their base in Tikrit. A month later, soldiers dropped him off at a local hospital. His family found him there four months later. Mr. Zoman was unconscious and being fed with a tube in his stomach. He had three skull fractures, a broken thumb, and burns on the soles of his feet. The Army had given the hospital a medical record, signed by Lieutenant Colonel Dr. Michael Hodges. It said that Mr. Zoman had suffered a heart attack and heatstroke; it did not mention the bruises, the lash and burn marks, or the fractures.[40]

Some clinicians resisted evaluating prisoners for abuse. An Abu Ghraib prisoner gave a detailed account of being beaten, having his head dunked in water, being butted against a wall, and being sodomized with a baton until he bled from his rectum. Two weeks after the alleged assault, an Army investigator took the prisoner to a physician, told the physician of the allegation, and requested a "medical examination specifically for trauma due to sodomy." The physician, who held the rank of colonel, did not examine the rectum but he nonetheless reported no signs of anal tearing.

The investigation was closed with a note by the investigating officer: "If there isn't medical evidence then this terrorist lied and you should find a way to charge him with perjury, filing a false statement and anything else available. That is the only way that these people will learn the value of their word and that there are consequences for a lack of integrity."[41]

Records can lie. At Camp Mercury in Iraq, guards regularly abused prisoners but a physician's assistant would record that the new injuries, including fractures, were present at capture, not acquired during imprisonment.[42] Some medical personnel offered far-fetched medical rationalizations for abusive treatment or injuries. Investigators at Mosul prison in Iraq obtained numerous sworn accounts of abuse while checking out a claim that a soldier had broken Salah Salih Jassim's jaw.[43] This imprisoned high school student was arrested along with his father, who had been an officer in Saddam Hussein's militia; he was not suspected of a crime.[44] The physician's note does not show any medical inquiry into how the jaw came to be fractured.[45] Neither the medic nor the physician looked for other bruises or removed the prisoner's shirt.[46–48] Later, the physician told investigators that the jaw might have been weakened by an unnoticed fracture in the past.[49] A prisoner at a secret prison near Baghdad was blindfolded and kept in isolation for sixteen days. He suffered a panic attack and screamed to be placed with other prisoners. The guards bound his wrists together and, for three hours, placed him between two stretchers that were tied together to form a human sandwich. A physician who held the rank of captain freed him but recorded that the panic attacks were "seizure like episodes," for which restraint between the stretchers was medically appropriate to prevent injuries. On that basis, investigators concluded that the guards "used justifiable means to control the prisoner during his seizures."[50]

Often, medical records were "lost" or went unsought. A physician who did postinterrogation physicals recalled that a prisoner had complained of being beaten; the physician said he did not see bruising and the medical record could not be found.[51] Investigators thought the complaint of a high-value Tikrit inmate of being chilled with an air conditioner and beaten, kicked, and dragged were credible, but they closed the investigation because neither the detaining soldiers nor the medical records could be found.[52] A Tikrit inmate described three days of beatings after which he had bloody urine but investigators could not find a medical record of his treatment.[53] Another Tikrit inmate had a long scalp laceration and multiple bruises apparently inflicted by Iraqi police before they turned him over to the Americans. That investigation was inconclusive, in part because medical logs were not kept.[54] In 2004, a woman prisoner at Abu Ghraib reported of being forced to crawl on concrete on her bare hands and knees, stripped in front of male soldiers and her nephew, and hit with a stick. The investigator's handwritten notes report her saying that she told two physicians of being beaten with a plastic chair that splintered and left a piece in her foot. A physician reportedly extracted a shard of the chair and gave her antibiotics. She said another physician told her that it "looks like you were run over by a guard" and to thank God that her brain was not injured. Investigators did not record any attempt to locate the medical records.[55]

"Lost" records were even used against an American soldier. In January 2003, Specialist Sean Baker put on a Guantánamo prisoner's uniform to allow an "internal reaction force" to practice extracting a prisoner from a cell. The extraction force was not told that Baker was an American. Baker recalls, "They grabbed my arms, my legs, twisted me up and . . . got up on my back from behind and put pressure down on me while I was face down." Guard Scott Sinclair "began to choke me and press my head against the floor." He twice "slammed my head against the floor and continued to choke me." Finally, the exercise was stopped. Baker was hospitalized with brain trauma and now suffers from seizures four times each week despite taking several anticonvulsants. The Guantánamo commander aborted an inquiry into Baker's injuries. The videotape of the training exercise was "lost." Eighteen months later, a Pentagon spokesperson, Major Laurie Arellano, told reporters that Baker's medical discharge was not related to his military duty. Baker then gave reporters a statement by an Army Physical Evaluation Board that had concluded that his injuries and disabilities were due to the beating. Major Arellano then conceded that the beatings were a factor in Baker's discharge, stating that she had new information about the medical evaluation.[56-58]

Some cases of abuse were dropped when a prisoner signed a document disavowing the allegations of abuse. For example, a medic recorded abrasions, bruises, a broken nose, and a fractured leg in a brief medical note that a physician signed without examining or interviewing the battered prisoner. The lack of a physician's note clearly harmed the case. The prisoner decided to drop his complaint and investigators accepted his formal statement: "I swear under oath that I do not want to file a complaint against the American Forces so I can get released."[59]

Sometimes passivity took the form of medically discharging a prisoner back to his or her abusers. A 2003 medical record tells of an Iraqi prisoner who was treated for a broken collarbone, a fracture of the bone below his eye, and pain in his left arm. After treatment, the prisoner was sent back to his cell.[60] There are many accounts of medical inattention to injuries from beatings at the detention center in Mosul, Iraq.[61] In one, a medic watched guards beat a prisoner and burn him by dragging him over hot stones. The prisoner was taken to the hospital, where he was treated by a physician, after which he was returned to the guards who had abused him. The investigation was closed because the physician did not sign the medical record and could not be identified.[62]

In this kind of environment, the assurance of silence apparently encouraged some medical personnel to collaborate in abusing prisoners. An intelligence officer at Na'ma in Iraq complained that a "medic aggressively ran to the detainee and ripped up the detainee's pants with a surgical scissors when the detainee was a little bit slow at responding to his command of 'take off your pants' " during an interrogation.[63] In November 2003, the guard Charles Graner lacerated an Abu Ghraib prisoner's face during a beating. A male medic came and allowed Graner to suture the wound while being photographed.[64–68] As Graner put it in an e-mail that he sent with the photograph, "Try doing this at home and they'll lock you up if you don't have some kind of license. . . . Not only was I the healer, I was the hurter."[69] The Army excused the medic because he told them that he believed Graner was trained to suture lacerations.[70] Perhaps so, but why is there another Abu Ghraib photograph showing a smiling woman guard suturing a prisoner's laceration? In a similar case, investigators recommended disciplining a guard who stepped on a prisoner's chest while the inmate was being sutured, but they did not censure the medic who allowed that abuse.[71] In Iraq, an anesthesiologist repeatedly dropped a two-pound bag of intravenous fluid on a patient, a nurse deliberately delayed giving pain medication, and medical staff fed pork to Muslim patients.[72] In a civil lawsuit, a Guantánamo prisoner says that a medic told guards to hit the head without hitting the eyes and that a nurse then refused to treat the wound the guards inflicted.[73]

Some accounts of abuse by clinicians are difficult to evaluate because it is possible that nonclinician soldiers presented themselves as medical personnel. Robert Hoyt, a U.S. physician, described plainclothes U.S. personnel commandeering a prison operating room to interview what they called "really bad guys." The interrogators used medical props. Dr. Hoyt and his colleagues heard shouting from the operating room and intervened to stop the misuse of medical facilities. He also saw an interrogator threaten an inpatient.[74]

Guantánamo is notable for a successful medical protest of prisoner abuse. In 2002, Dr. Michael Gelles, the chief psychologist of the Navy Criminal Investigative Service, complained about "abusive techniques" to the Navy's general counsel, Alberto Mora. Mora took the matter to the highest level of the Pentagon, asserting that the techniques were "unlawful and unworthy of the military services." Senior Navy officials were so upset by Gelles's reports that they considered pulling out of the Guantánamo interrogations. Secretary of Defense Rumsfeld responded by revoking his initial list of approved interrogation techniques; he issued a more tempered list in April 2003.[75]

THE RED CROSS

The International Committee of the Red Cross (ICRC) is a special kind of human rights organization. Its extraordinary access to prisons is possible because its reports go exclusively to prison authorities and are not publicly issued.[76] They may not even be subpoenaed for war crimes trials. In this way, the ICRC differs from organizations like Amnesty International and Human Rights Watch that issue public reports on prison conditions and human rights abuses.

The ICRC tried to curtail abuses at American prisons in Iraq, in Afghanistan, and at Guantánamo. At Guantánamo, it presented its concerns to senior officers at sixteen classified meetings between November 2002 and mid-April 2003.[77] Those meetings reportedly broke off in the fall of 2003 partly over Red Cross objections to interrogators' access to the medical records of prisoners. In Afghanistan, the ICRC protested the practice of suspending prisoners, as was done to Dilawar shortly before he died. In mid-2003, the Red Cross submitted to the Defense Department a list of two hundred allegations of mistreatment of Iraqi prisoners. Two months later, it sent fifty more complaints from Baghdad's Camp Cropper alone. A Red Cross medical monitor saw a prisoner with bruises on his back, blood in his urine, and a broken rib, findings consistent with the prisoner's report as to how he was beaten for threatening to complain to the ICRC. The Red Cross also saw burns on a sixty-one-year-old Camp Bucca prisoner who told of being forced to sit on the hot hood of a vehicle until he lost consciousness.[78] The Red Cross protested the Army's decision to deny it access to Abu Ghraib prisoners under interrogation. The ICRC said that this denial violated "International Humanitarian Law" as well as the Third (Prisoners of War) and Fourth (Civilian Persons in Time of War) Geneva Conventions.[79]

In 2004, the Red Cross gave the Army a summary of its 2003 visits to prisons in Iraq. That report was leaked to the press, to the ICRC's great displeasure. It described many seriously injured and abused prisoners and concluded that persons suspected of security offenses or believed to have intelligence value were at "high risk of being subjected to a variety of harsh treatments which in some cases was tantamount to torture in order to force cooperation with their interrogators."[80] Local commanders minimized or professed to disbelieve ICRC allegations, and they denied the ICRC's requests to visit and monitor prisoners in many locations.[81]

MEDICAL SOCIETIES

U.S. medical societies were unprepared for the possibility that American military medical personnel might be complicit with prisoner abuse and neglect. The American Medical Association (AMA) kept a low profile as concern over medical complicity with abuses of prisoners mounted. Its 250,000 members include somewhat less than a third of American physicians and a large contingent of physicians with military backgrounds. In addition, AMA lobbyists were focused on a bill setting Medicare reimbursements to physicians and another bill to limit malpractice lawsuits and awards. The latter issue is a very strong predictor of AMA lobbying priorities.[82]

The 120,000 internists of the American College of Physicians (ACP) were much more aggressive. Ten years earlier, the ACP had differed with the AMA and supported President Clinton's health-care reform effort. In October 2003, six months before the Abu Ghraib photographs surfaced, the ACP president wrote President Bush, expressing concern about reported abuses of prisoners. The ACP did not receive a reply. An ACP official grounded the college's concern in its 1993 policy paper, which states:

> The key to an effective response to torture lies in concerted action on the part of the medical profession. Physicians, regardless of their specialty and the way in which they express their medical skills on a daily basis, respond to torture through their affiliations with the medical profession. Medical associations can expand and magnify the effectiveness of an individual physician's work.[83]

The ACP sent another letter to President Bush in May 2004, after the Abu Ghraib photographs became public. That summer, it failed to persuade the AMA to support a call for independent investigations of prisoner abuse. The AMA did endorse and offered to assist the Department of Defense's own internal investigations.[84,85]

During the summer of 2004, *The New England Journal of Medicine* and the British medical journal *The Lancet* published articles claiming that American military medical personnel were complicit with prisoner abuse.[86,87] The British Medical Association, the British Medical Foundation for the Care of Victims of Torture, and the American Medical Student Association (which is not part of the AMA) called on the AMA to investigate and discipline physicians who abetted the abuses.[88] Dr.

Matthew Wynia, director of the AMA Institute for Ethics, affirmed the organization's pre–Abu Ghraib position on physicians and torture:

> Physicians must oppose and must not participate in torture for any reason. Participation in torture includes, but is not limited to, providing or withholding any services, substances or knowledge to facilitate the practice of torture. Physicians must not be present when torture is used or threatened. Physicians may treat prisoners or detainees if doing so is in their best interest, but physicians should not treat individuals to verify their health so that torture can begin or continue. Physicians who treat torture victims should not be persecuted.[89]

Dr. Wynia cited Major General George Fay's investigation of intelligence abuses at Abu Ghraib, which found that two prison medics did not report abuse and added that several physicians did "the right thing under adverse circumstances."[90]

Even AMA medical publications, which are editorially independent from the organization, did not publish articles on prison human rights abuses until late 2005.[91,92] Their silence contrasts with the record of the *British Medical Journal, The Lancet, Surgery, Science, The New England Journal of Medicine, MedScape*, and the *Annals of Plastic Surgery*, as well as the intense concern in the lay media on this matter.

A year after the release of the Abu Ghraib photographs, American medical societies were finally mobilized by the appearance of an American Psychological Association report, large hunger strikes at Guantánamo Bay, and an attempt by Senator John McCain (R-Arizona) to attach a ban on government torture to a defense appropriations bill.[93] By mid-2005, the AMA was treading water. Likewise, the American Psychiatric Association tepidly opined that it was "troubled by recent reports regarding alleged violations of professional medical ethics by psychiatrists at Guantanamo Bay," but it did not call for an investigation, define ethics rules for psychiatrists who were asked to participate in interrogation, or even mention Iraq or Afghanistan.[94]

In June 2005, the American Psychological Association released a report by a presidential task force, "Psychological Ethics and National Security." The ensuing debate revealed the fault lines between medical ethics and coercive interrogations. The association had created the task force to develop standards for military psychologists who assisted with interrogations. Its report began solidly enough by asserting that the United Nations Convention Against Torture and Other Cruel, Inhuman or Degrading Treatment or Punishment and the Geneva Convention Relative to the Treatment of Prisoners of War applied to all prisoners. It also said that with regard to "cruel, inhuman or degrading treatment," psychologists "have an ethical responsibility to report these acts to the appropriate authorities." The task force then diverged from international codes of medical ethics by endorsing the Defense Department's position that psychologists working with interrogators could use information from medical records to help ensure that the interrogation "remains safe," if that information was not used to the "detriment of the individual's safety and well being."[95] The association's report left open the possibility that a psychologist might conceal his or her professional identity or relationship with interrogators from a prisoner, an apparent violation of its own ethics code.

Human rights advocates assailed the association's report.[96,97] Physicians for Human Rights said that it violated World Medical Association guidelines, authorized psychologists' collaboration in illegal coercive interrogations, and violated the association's own confidentiality code.[98] These are troubling charges, which suggest that the association accommodated the Defense Department's belittling of the long-term harms of coercive interrogations, the dangers of breaching medical confidentiality, and the medical harms that could ensue if prisoners did not trust and speak freely with their clinicians. The task force's makeup was also criticized.[99] Six of ten members, as described by the association, had military or intelligence backgrounds; most of these had overseen activities or personnel at Guantánamo Bay or Iraq:

- Colonel Morgan Banks, Ph.D., is chief of the Psychological Applications Directorate of the U.S. Army Special Operations Command, is responsible for operational psychology support to Special Operations combat units, and provides consultation on interrogation. In 2001, he worked at Bagram in Afghanistan supporting combat operations against Al Qaeda and Taliban fighters.

- Robert Fein, Ph.D., is a forensic psychologist who consults for the Directorate for Behavioral Sciences of the Department of Defense Counterintelligence Field Activity and other agencies.

- Michael Gelles, Psy.D., is the chief psychologist for the Naval Criminal Investigative Service, where he conducts psychological assessments of criminals and victims. He called attention to abusive interrogations at Guantánamo.

- Colonel Larry James, Ph.D., was chief psychologist for the Joint Intelligence Group at Guantánamo Bay in 2003. He then became director of the Behavioral Science Unit at Abu Ghraib, where he was responsible for developing legal and ethical policies consistent with the Geneva Convention in response to the abuse scandal.

- Captain Bryce Lefever, Ph.D., is a clinical psychologist whose career is with Navy operations pertaining to interrogation.

- R. Scott Shumate, Psy.D., is director of behavioral science for counterintelligence field activity at the Department of Defense, where he oversees risk assessments of Guantánamo Bay detainees.

Four members, including the nonvoting chair, were unaffiliated with the Defense Department.

- Jean Maria Arrigo, Ph.D., is an academic expert on torture and interrogation.

- Olivia Moorehead-Slaughter, Ph.D., is on the Massachusetts licensing board for psychologists and on the APA's ethics committee.

- Nina Thomas, Ph.D., is a psychologist with expertise in treating trauma and disaster victims.

- Michael Wessells, Ph.D., is past president of the Division of Peace Psychology of the American Psychological Association and of Psychologists for Social Responsibility.

Although the association needed military expertise to knowledgeably address its subject matter, it is unclear why it gave military officers, many of whom had worked at the epicenter of the controversial programs, six of nine votes on the task force. It could have called these experts as nonvoting witnesses. It could have recruited senior and long retired military intelligence officials. It could have brought on voting human rights experts to balance the vote and reduce the conflict of interest. Instead, it compromised the impartiality and credibility of its task force.

Four months after the American Psychological Association report and after pressure from Physicians for Human Rights, the psychiatrist Robert Lifton, and others, the American Psychiatric Association stiffened its position and succinctly rejected the American Psychological Association's view: "Our position is very direct; psychiatrists should not participate on these biscuit [BSCT: Behavioral Science Consultation] teams."[100]

In September 2005, Senator John McCain, a Republican Vietnam-era veteran and former POW and torture victim, proposed to amend a defense appropriations bill to bar government agencies from treating prisoners in a "cruel, inhuman, or degrading manner." President Bush vowed to veto such language and Vice President Cheney led the administration's effort to defeat the amendment, an effort that led the disgusted former CIA director Stansfield Turner to say, "I'm embarrassed the United States has a vice president for torture. . . . He condones torture, what else is he?"[101] Three weeks before the Senate vote, the American College of Physicians publicly urged the McCain amendment's passage.[102] The Senate voted 90 to 9 in favor of the amendment. Three weeks *after* the vote, when the bill was en route to a less certain fate in the House of Representatives, the AMA quietly wrote to a Senate committee supporting the McCain amendment.[103] It did not issue a press release or post the letter on its website. The American Psychiatric Association and the American Psychological Association publicly urged passage of the McCain amendment.[104]

In November, AMA delegates endorsed a motion by the American Academy of Child and Adolescent Psychiatry and the American Academy of Pediatrics asking the AMA to delineate interrogation ethics standards for physicians.[105] The AMA has not called for an independent investigation of the prison medical system. It has not exercised an option in its own rules that would enable it to convene a special investigative jury to evaluate either the phenomenon as a whole or specific physicians who may have acted unprofessionally.

Other American health societies have spoken in various ways. The American Public Health Association condemned participation by health professionals in abuse or torture and urged that they report abuses.[106] The American Nursing Association's president wrote to Major General Gale Pollock, head of the Army Nurse Corps, who replied that there was no evidence of Army Nurse Corps members being involved in any inappropriate or unethical behavior.[107] The board of the American Society for Bioethics and Humanities asked President Bush to empower an independent investigation of medical activities and to commission standards for health professionals' conduct.[108] In response to my inquiries, the American Association for Correctional and Forensic Psychology, the American Correctional Health Services Association, the National Arab American Medical Association, the National Medical Association, and the Society of Correctional Physicians state that they have not taken any action.

Medical human rights groups have been much more aggressive. Physicians for Human Rights releases reports, issues letters (including a harsh letter from former president George H. W. Bush's physician[109]), maintains an active website, and has set up a petition for medical leaders to call for an independent investigation of the abuses and for reform to prevent further abuses.[110] The World Medical Association (WMA), a congress of national medical societies, asserted that physicians have the same professional duty to refrain from complicity with torture during war as they have during peace or civil unrest. The WMA also strengthened its position condemning medical collaboration in coercive interrogation.[111,112] Other human rights groups, especially Human Rights Watch, Human Rights First, and Amnesty International, have issued numerous reports about the abuses of prisoners, some of which address health-related issues. Centers for treating torture victims, such as the Center for Victims of Torture in Minneapolis, are also speaking out on this matter.

THE DEFENSE DEPARTMENT RESPONDS

The Defense Department rejects allegations that military medical personnel passively acquiesced to prisoner abuse. In 2004, Major General Fay's investigation found that medical personnel cited only two Abu Ghraib medics as having "observed and failed to report instances of abuse."[113] The office of the Army Inspector General has not declassified a survey it undertook asking medical officers in Afghanistan and Iraq whether they reported abuses or instructed their subordinates to report abuses.[114] In February 2005, Dr. William Winkenwerder said that the Defense Department was aware of only five to seven incidents "principally involving medics" who did not report abuse that they observed.[115] A month later, Admiral Church concluded that it was impossible to assess "whether medical personnel serving the Global War on Terror have adequately discharged their obligation to report (and where possible prevent) detainee abuse. However, our interviews with medical personnel indicate that they had only infrequently suspected or witnessed abuse and had in those instances reported it through the chain of command."[116]

A month later, the Army Surgeon General attempted to lay the matter to rest. Citing his office's own survey, he claimed that only 5 percent of 1,200 medical personnel who served in Iraq, in Afghanistan, or at Guantánamo during the peak period of abuse said that prisoners had reported being abused.[117] Remarkably, not one of the clinicians surveyed by the Army Surgeon General reported seeing actual or suspected abuse of any prisoner in Afghanistan.[118] The explanation for this finding may lie in how readily the Surgeon General's researchers accepted "see no evil" answers.

Investigation records are more worrisome. Army medic Robert Melone, with the 772nd MP Company at Bagram prison in Afghanistan, reported that three prisoners told him that they had been abused by U.S. soldiers and that they bore signs of being abused. However, by the time investigators interviewed him after the torture deaths of Dilawar and

Habibullah, Melone denied any knowledge of abuse except for seeing prisoners handcuffed with their arms elevated.[119] He recalled a guard coming to his tent one night and asking for help for Habibullah, who had stopped breathing. Melone replied, "What are you getting me for?" and told the guard to call an ambulance. He says he heard later that the prisoner died after being beaten and suspended. He could not recall anything about Dilawar, who also died while he was on call.

An intelligence soldier at the prison in Kandahar, Afghanistan, described a medical exam during which a large MP, not the clinician, lubricated two of his fingers to perform the rectal exam. "Without warning the EPW [enemy prisoner of war], and in a cruel way, he pushed both his fingers into the EPW's anus. This caused the EPW to scream and fall to the ground violently."[120] A military translator, also at Kandahar, testified how prisoners repeatedly complained of abuse to a physician who held the rank of captain and to a medic who "both made comments to the effect that they, the detainees, wouldn't hurt if they didn't get hit and to tell them not to get hit again. These two individuals did not want to give pain medicine to these particular detainees."[121]

According to the Army Surgeon General, medical personnel "aggressively reported actual and suspected detainee abuse to the proper authorities."[122] However, it was FBI, not medical personnel, who led the protest against abusive and injurious treatment at Guantánamo.[123,124] After the Abu Ghraib scandal became public, clinicians became more willing to admit seeing abuse. A quarter told military surveyors that they had seen prisoners who had reported being abused, although few said they saw signs of injuries.

The Surgeon General's researchers found that 34 of 463 clinic records noted either suspected abuse or an allegation of abuse, but only 10 of those charts recorded any action taken to address the abuse.[125] However, the researchers ignored records describing traumatic injuries that were simply diagnosed and treated without any comment on how the injury was acquired. One such record was that of the young prisoner with a broken jaw, who was discussed earlier.[126]

The Surgeon General's study is vague on critical points as well. It does not tell how many of the records examined came from large prisons or from remote operating bases where abuse was more easily concealed. It does not discuss the fact that its researchers could not have examined many classified preinterrogation and postinterrogation medical exams, which were kept apart from routine medical records. Surgeon General Kiley accepted the assessment of his investigator, Major General Lester Martinez-Lopez, M.D., M.P.H.: "By any measure, medical personnel were exceptionally vigilant in reporting actual or suspected detainee abuse."[127]

The Army Surgeon General did find poor medical policies for addressing prisoner abuse. There was no definition of abuse in Army medical regulations or training in abuse reporting until after the Abu Ghraib scandal had surfaced. The armed forces did not teach medical soldiers the UN rules that oblige medical officers to report situations where prison treatment has injured prisoners. Policies for reporting abuse differed by branch of service and theater of operation.[128] This murky policy climate did not deter Abu Ghraib investigators from asserting that clinicians must report prisoner abuse.[129] Major General Fay wrote,

> The duty to report detainee abuse is closely tied to the duty to protect. The failure to report an abusive incident could result in additional abuse. Soldiers who witness these offenses have an obligation to report the violations under the provision of Article 92, UCMJ [Uniform Code of Military Justice]. Soldiers who are informed of such abuses also have a duty to report violations. Depending on their positions and their assigned duties, the failure to report detainee abuse could support a charge of dereliction of duty, a violation of Article 92 of the Uniform Code of Military Justice.[130]

Few clinicians would read Article 92 as describing a duty to report prisoner abuse or neglect:

> Any person who (1) Violates or fails to obey any lawful general order or regulation; (2) Having knowledge of any other lawful order issued by any member of the armed forces, which it is his duty to obey, fails to

obey the order; or (3) Is derelict in the performance of his duties; shall be punished as a court-martial may direct.

DISCUSSION

Silence can be personal or institutional. A clinician may passively watch a prisoner being abused or may fail to document a patient's injuries or allegations. A pathologist who has conducted an autopsy on a fatally beaten prisoner may remain silent after a government spokesperson untruthfully states that the death resulted from natural causes. A military medical command may fail to protest as its prisoners receive inadequate food, medications, sanitation, and protection from mortar and sniper fire. A civilian medical society may fail to call for an independent and transparent investigation when prisoners' health and the profession's stature are harmed by medical complicity with abuses.

Silence was the policy and practice in U.S. prisons. Two experienced interrogators at a Baghdad prison saw beaten and burned prisoners and watched an MP punch a prisoner in the face, after which the prisoner's medical care went deliberately unrecorded. They presented a formal complaint to their commander, who confiscated the photographs of the injured prisoner, threatened them, took their vehicle keys, confined them to base, ordered them not to talk to anyone in the United States, and told them that their e-mail would be monitored. Those interrogators went outside of their chain of command to prompt an investigation.[131] Officers told prison medical staff in Iraq and Guantánamo not to talk about their experiences and impressions.[132] An intelligence specialist, Samual Provance, was demoted, lost his security clearance, and was assigned to guard duty picking up trash after protesting the abuses at Abu Ghraib and the subsequent effort to confine the investigations to the culpability of low-ranking guards.[133] Likewise, a medic reported "a lot of peer pressure to keep one's mouth shut and 'do what they do.' "[134] As a senior military interrogator put it, "If you saw something and reported it, it was your word against theirs. The discipline [for abusers] was a slap on the hand."[135]

The silence of prison health care providers had terrible consequences.

It allowed abuses to continue and to go unpunished. It resulted in the return of abused prisoners to abusive guards. It reinforced the breakdown in command accountability, an atmosphere in which abuse flourishes. Prisoners lost the physician as a human rights advocate. They lost a confidant to whom they could disclose depression, anxiety, or stress disorders that set the stage for riots, suicide attempts, and disabling post-traumatic stress disorder. Mistrustful prisoners may fail to disclose medical symptoms that signify diseases like tuberculosis, which can infect other prisoners or guards. As the Red Cross put it, the Guantánamo "prisoners lost trust in the physicians."[136]

The duty to report abused patients appears at several points in medical ethics. In all states, clinicians must report even the suspicion that a child has been abused. In many states, similar laws mandate reports when the patient is a vulnerable adult. The duty of prison clinicians with regard to abused prisoners is still being articulated. Amnesty International "calls on health professionals witnessing torture or other cruel, inhuman or degrading treatment or punishment, or the effects of such violations, to report their observations to their immediate manager and to their professional association." The British Medical Association supports clear reporting procedures with policies to protect whistleblowers from reprisals.[137]

It requires courage for a nurse, a physician, or a medical society to practice ethical medicine when feeling caught between conflicting duties. Most such "dual loyalty" situations arise when the duty to a patient's well-being conflicts with a powerful organization's interest.[138] For example, a company might pressure physicians not to report hazards, such as the asbestos lung injuries that afflicted shipbuilders. Drug companies coerce researchers to underplay side effects. Military physicians or nurses may feel pressured to acquiesce to, or assist in, abusive interrogations. Military pathologists may feel that they should not dissent when they hear military spokespeople assert that a murdered prisoner died of natural causes. A medical society may want to avoid alienating political allies whom it needs to advance its main policy priorities.

In general, the interests of patients, corporations, and nations are best served when health professionals individually and collectively advocate for health. Occupational physicians who push back against shipyard owners create safer workplaces. Researchers who resist a drug company's desire to spin research findings create better drugs. Medical opposition to concealing homicide or harsh interrogations would have better served the health interests of prisoners and prevented enormous damage to the reputation of the United States and its armed forces. The voice of medicine matters.

A prison medical staff is the front line of torture prevention. Unlike Red Cross monitors, doctors, nurses, and medics are in nearly all prisons at nearly all times.[139] They see most, if not all, prisoners. They are most likely to witness abuse or neglect. They are most likely to see signs of abuse before the bruises heal. Prison medical professionals and their counterparts in civilian society must choose to acquiesce or oppose, to be accomplices or healers.

Domestic medical societies also must choose. They are a respected domestic constituency and belong to an honored international community. Mere endorsement of antitorture guidelines is not enough. The failure of U.S. medical societies to collectively and forcefully press for release of the classified appendices of the investigations of the medical services, and for an independent, empowered, and transparent investigation of medical complicity in prisoner neglect and abuse may have been decisive in allowing the government to deflect similar appeals by smaller human rights organizations. Medical participation in human rights abuses stained the profession. Silence allowed the stain to spread and set.

PART III
"PLAIN LANGUAGE"

The President should know that a decision that the Conventions do apply is consistent with the plain language of the Conventions and the unvaried practice of the United States in introducing its forces into conflict over fifty years.

WILLIAM H. TAFT IV,
legal advisor, U.S. Department of State

CHAPTER 7

GRAVE BREACHES

THE ABUSE AND NEGLECT OF PRISONERS IN THE WAR ON TERROR were not the isolated acts of a few soldiers. They were not limited to a few brief or local breakdowns in command authority. This book has shown that events similar to those photographed at Abu Ghraib in late 2003 occurred at Guantánamo and in prisons scattered across Iraq and Afghanistan. This book is confined by its focus on armed forces and CIA files pertaining to medical personnel; less restricted reviews will find similar mistreatment at an even larger number of prisons. Even those broader investigations will be unable to examine secret prisons operated on behalf of the U.S. government in Africa, Europe, and Asia. The large scale of the abuses raises a large-scale question: if the medical abuse and neglect of prisoners was not a matter of isolated criminal acts or exceptional command failures, did it arise from government policy?

To assess that question, several issues must be explored. Can the policy foundation for the abuses be identified? Were policy makers aware of other policy options, and were such options rejected? Are the policy makers potentially responsible for war crimes?

THE POLICY FOUNDATION OF ABUSE

U.S. government officials created the prison medical system in three steps.

1. Void preexisting standards for the treatment of prisoners, such as the Geneva Conventions and the United States' own War Crimes Act.

2. Create new policies that risk prison human rights violations.

3. Implement the new prison policies and allow those consequences to unfold.

STEP 1: VOID PREEXISTING PRISON STANDARDS

The United States invaded Afghanistan in October 2001, soon after the attacks of September 11. It began taking prisoners immediately. Guantánamo Bay received its first prisoners in January 2002. The Bush administration quickly sought to void the applicability of the Geneva Conventions and the U.S. War Crimes Act for Al Qaeda and Taliban prisoners. The War Crimes Act is a federal law, which makes breaking the Geneva Conventions or other international laws a federal crime.[1]

> (a) Offense. Whoever, whether inside or outside the United States, commits a war crime, in any of the circumstances described in subsection (b), shall be fined under this title or imprisoned for life or any term of years, or both, and if death results to the victim, shall also be subject to the penalty of death.
>
> (b) Circumstances. The circumstances referred to in subsection (a) are that the person committing such war crime . . . is a member of the Armed Forces of the United States or a national of the United States.
>
> (c) Definition. As used in this section the term "war crime" means any conduct: (1) defined as a grave breach in any of the international conventions signed at Geneva 12 August 1949, or any protocol to such convention to which the United States is a party; . . . (3) which constitute a violation of common Article 3 of the international conventions signed at Geneva.

Lawyers at the Justice Department and Defense Department soon produced memos concluding that the Geneva Conventions and the War Crimes Act did not apply to Al Qaeda, because it was not a nation, or to the Taliban, because Afghanistan was a "failed state" by virtue of being controlled by Al Qaeda.[2-4] Justice Department lawyers said that the president's constitutional war-making power allowed him to suspend the conventions and the War Crimes Act.[5] On January 19, 2002, Secretary of Defense Rumsfeld sent the following memo to the chairman of the Joint Chiefs of Staff:

> The United States has determined that Al Qaida and Taliban individuals under the control of the Department of Defense are not entitled to prisoner of war status for purposes of the Geneva Convention of 1949. . . .
> [T]reat them humanely and, to the extent appropriate and consistent with military necessity, in a manner consistent with the principles of the Geneva Conventions of 1949.[6]

The date, January 19, is worth noting. Secretary Rumsfeld sent this memo before the Justice Department and Defense Department memos were finalized and three weeks before the president issued his executive order asserting that the Geneva Conventions did not apply to Taliban or Al Qaeda prisoners.

Secretary of State Colin Powell and State Department Counsel Howard Taft IV dissented from the views emerging from the Departments of Justice and Defense. As they expressed their concerns, they did not know that Secretary of Defense Rumsfeld had already voided the Geneva Conventions. On January 26, 2002, Secretary of State Powell wrote a scathing letter to the president's lawyer arguing in favor of honoring the Geneva Conventions. He argued that revoking the conventions would

> reverse over a century of U.S. policy and practice in supporting the Geneva conventions and undermine the protections of the law of war for our troops, both in this specific conflict and in general.
> [Revocation] has a high cost in terms of negative international reaction. . . .
> It will undermine public support among critical allies, making military cooperation more difficult to sustain.
> Europeans and others will likely have legal problems with extradition or other form of cooperation in law enforcement, including in bringing terrorists to justice.

It may provoke some individual foreign prosecutors to investigate and prosecute our officials and troops.

It will . . . deprive us of important legal options.[7]

On February 2, Howard Taft wrote,

The President should know that a decision that the Conventions do apply is consistent with the plain language of the Conventions and the unvaried practice of the United States in introducing its forces into conflict over fifty years. . . .

A decision that the Conventions do not apply to the conflict in Afghanistan . . . deprives our troops there of any claim to the protection of the Conventions in the event they are captured and weakens the protections accorded by the Conventions to our troops in future conflicts.[8]

The Taft and Powell memos prudently discussed how the United States' security needs could be met within the framework of international law. The choice to conform to human rights law was possible; that choice was rejected. Then–Attorney General John Ashcroft and the White House legal counsel, Alberto Gonzales, who succeeded Ashcroft in 2005, dismissed the arguments of the State Department officials.[9,10]

On February 7, President Bush signed an executive order that directly used Secretary Rumsfeld's January 19 language,

Article 3 of Geneva does not apply to either al-Qaida or Taliban detainees. . . .

As a matter of policy, the United States Armed Forces shall continue to treat detainees humanely and, to the extent appropriate and consistent with military necessity, in a manner consistent with the principles of Geneva.[11]

The president's directive deferred to the principles, rather than the provisions, of the Geneva Conventions. He subordinated the Geneva standards to an undefined "military necessity." He never limited the coercion of prisoners to "ticking time bomb" criteria. Soon, the words "appropriate and consistent with military necessity" became the sardonic and unchallengeable catechism of abusive guards at Guantánamo.[12]

In setting aside the Geneva Conventions, the administration addressed prisoners' medical care only in passing. The attorney general's office advised the White House and Defense Department that "difficulty in meeting all of the conditions set for POW camp conditions" was not a grave breach of the Geneva Conventions.[13] "Grave breaches" of the conventions, by definition, violate the U.S. War Crimes Act. In a section entitled "Justified Deviations from Geneva Convention Requirements," the assistant attorney general, Jay Bybee, wrote that since Guantánamo prisoners were being housed in "basic humane conditions, are not being physically mistreated and are receiving medical care," the War Crimes Act was not being violated.[14] That legal opinion seems to concede that inhumane conditions, mistreatment, or inadequate medical care could constitute a grave breach of the conventions and therefore violate the War Crimes Act.

The old rules were now cleared. The administration could now write its own policies.

STEP 2: CREATE NEW PRISON MEDICAL STANDARDS

In August 2002, six months after President Bush set aside the Geneva Conventions for Afghanistan and Guantánamo prisoners, the Justice and Defense Departments began to work on coercive interrogation policies. Justice Department attorneys took the lead, claiming that the president's constitutional power to wage war, gather intelligence, and protect national security could not be constrained by the UN's Convention Against Torture and Other Cruel, Inhuman or Degrading Treatment or Punishment and the U.S. Torture Victims Treatment Act of 1987. They also argued that the definition of torture in United States federal law was vague.[15–17] They went further, offering a novel distinction between torture and cruel treatment and defining physical torture as so severe that it must seem to threaten life itself.

> [W]e conclude that torture . . . covers only extreme acts. Severe pain is generally of the kind difficult for the victim to endure. Where the pain

is physical, it must be of an intensity akin to that which accompanies serious physical injury such as death or organ failure. Severe mental pain requires suffering not just at the moment of infliction but it also requires lasting psychological harm, such as seen in mental disorders like posttraumatic stress disorder. . . . Because the acts inflicting torture are extreme, there is significant range of actions that though they might constitute cruel, inhuman, or degrading treatment or punishment fail to rise to the level of torture.

Three months later, Guantánamo commanders asked for permission to apply the new latitude in their interrogations.

Lieutenant Colonel Jerald Phifer, the commander of Guantánamo interrogation teams, sent a memo to Major General Michael Dunleavy, the commander of Joint Task Force 170, which was responsible for intelligence gathering at the prison. Phifer complained, "The current guidelines for interrogation procedures at GTMO [Guantánamo] limit the ability of interrogators to counter advanced resistance."[18] General Dunleavy seconded Phifer's memo and forwarded it to the United States Southern Command in Miami.[19] Two weeks later, General James T. Hill, commander of the Southern Command, wrote to the Joint Chiefs of Staff, "Despite our best efforts, some detainees have tenaciously resisted our current interrogation methods. . . . I firmly believe that we must quickly provide Joint Task Force 170 [at Guantánamo] counter-resistance techniques to maximize the value of our intelligence collection mission."[20]

Lieutenant Colonel Diane Beaver, an attorney with Joint Task Force 170, proposed a medical role in harsh interrogations. She wrote that death threats, "exposure to cold weather or water is permissible with appropriate medical monitoring. The use of a wet towel to induce the misperception of suffocation would also be permissible if not done with the specific intent to cause prolonged mental harm and absent medical evidence that it would."[21] Secretary Rumsfeld approved Beaver's outline in November 2002, adding that the officer in charge of interrogation for detainees in isolation could reject or "approve all contacts with the detainee, to include medical visits of a non-emergent nature."[22] This latter provision was revoked because it clearly abrogated a detainee's right to request a medical evaluation.[23]

Secretary of Defense Rumsfeld then appointed a working group to develop interrogation policy.[24,25] The Defense Department working group essentially accepted the Department of Justice position on the legality of harsh interrogations. However, it did review military experience with coercive interrogation. It told Secretary Rumsfeld that "interrogation experts view the use of force as an inferior technique that yields information of questionable quality" and that has "adverse effects on future interrogations." The working group also said that using coercion might damage the admissibility of evidence, harm public support for the military effort, and endanger Americans who become POWs.[26] It warned: "Participation by US military personnel in interrogations which use techniques that are more aggressive than those appropriate for POWs would constitute a significant departure from traditional US military norms and could have an adverse impact on the cultural self-image of US military forces."[27] The group implicitly accepted medical collaboration with harsh interrogation, for it discussed using mind-altering drugs and the need for the "presence or availability (as appropriate) of qualified medical personnel."[28] It did not mention medical ethics codes or the history of medicine and prisoner abuse.

Upon receiving the working group's reports, Secretary Rumsfeld approved "counterresistance" interrogation techniques, including isolation, interrogation for twenty hours, deprivation of light and sound, and the use of loud sounds.[29] He noted that some nations might view these methods as inhumane, intimidating, or coercive, or as violating the Geneva Convention, but he asserted that the "provisions of the Geneva Convention are not applicable" to Guantánamo detainees.[30]

The secretary's directive sketched a philosophy of a medical partnership with coercive interrogation: "Interrogations must always be planned, deliberate actions that take into account . . . a detainee's emotional and physical strengths and weaknesses. Interrogation approaches are designed to manipulate the detainee's emotions and weaknesses to gain his willing cooperation."[31] Secretary Rumsfeld proposed three clinical roles in interrogations. First, "The use of isolation as an interrogation technique requires detailed implementation instructions, including . . . medical and psychological review."[32] Second, "Application of these interrogation techniques is subject to the following general safeguards: . . . (iii) the detainee is medically and operationally evaluated as suitable (considering all techniques to be used in combination)."[33] Third, the secretary required "reasonable safeguards . . . [including] the presence or availability of qualified medical personnel."[34] Furthermore, Rumsfeld's proposal that interrogation plans coercively "manipulate the detainee's emotions and weaknesses" implicitly invited employing medical information for interrogative purposes. Secretary Rumsfeld's interrogation policy was now ready to pass down the chain of command to Guantánamo and Afghanistan.

Step 3: Implement the New Harsh Interrogation Policies

Rumsfeld's vision of medically vetted, medically informed, medically monitored interrogations was fleshed out in Army prisons. Major General Geoffrey Miller had assumed command of intelligence collection at Guantánamo in November 2002. He added Behavioral Science Consultation Teams and it is reasonable to surmise that he secured their access to clinical records. The medical interrogation policy trail from the Pentagon to Afghanistan is still classified, but it is clear that the practices followed Rumsfeld's model. Captain Carolyn Wood, who had a senior role in intelligence collection at Bagram prison in Afghanistan, brought the Bagram "Interrogation Rules of Engagement" to Abu Ghraib.[35] (See Chapter 3, "Interrogation," Figure 3.2.) Those rules reiterate the core Rumsfeld policy in their statement "Wounded or medically burdened detainees must be medically cleared prior to interrogation" and their provision for "Dietary Manip (monitored by med)."[36] Interrogators in Afghanistan had access to medical records but did not have a Behavioral Science Consultation Team.[37,38]

About four months after the Guantánamo and Afghanistan interrogation policies were implemented, Secretary Rumsfeld sent them to Iraq in August 2003. With the approval of the Joint Chiefs of Staff, he ordered Stephen Cambone, his undersecretary for intelligence, to improve military intelligence in Iraq.[39] Cambone, who had no background in intelligence, passed Rumsfeld's directive to General William "Jerry" Boykin. General Boykin, a Defense Department deputy undersecretary for intelligence, gives "holy war" speeches in uniform to civic and church groups on behalf of the "Faith Force Multiplier." As he puts it, "Satan wants to destroy this nation . . . and he wants to destroy us as a Christian army." Speaking of a captive Muslim fighter, Boykin says, "I knew that my God was bigger than his. I knew that my God was a real God and his was an idol." Boykin also knows that God chose George Bush to be president: "Why is this man in the White House? The majority of Americans did not vote for him. . . . [He is] in the White House because God put him there for a time such as this."[40] Boykin picked General Miller to carry Rumsfeld's model from Guantánamo to Iraq. That trip to Iraq and the designation of Abu Ghraib as an interrogation center are described in Chapter 3, "Interrogation." General Ricardo Sanchez, the commander of U.S. forces in Iraq, copied Secretary Rumsfeld's medical rules for interrogations verbatim.[41]

Secretary Rumsfeld created a new kind of Army interrogation system in Iraq, in Afghanistan, and at Guantánamo. The Joint Integration and Debriefing Centers, like Abu Ghraib, integrated interrogators and guards to exploit prisoners' weaknesses. Major General George Fay's investigation concluded this was a "nondoctrinal" organization, meaning that there were no policies to describe the governance of a dual-function interrogation center.[42] Provost Marshal Donald Ryder and Major Generals George Fay and Antonio Taguba agreed that the new centers' staff worked without clear policies and outside of a single command.[43,44] To make matters worse, neither interrogators nor guards were seasoned intelligence operatives. General Fay found that frontline staff had "no formal advanced interrogation training" in prisons. He also wrote that "with very few exceptions, combined Military Intelligence and Military Police training on the conduct of detainee operations is nonexistent."[45] In this rump interrogation system, clinicians performed preinterrogation physicals, supplied interrogators with medical information about prisoners, worked with Behavioral Science Consultation Teams to design interrogation plans, and monitored or terminated harsh interrogations.

GRAVE BREACHES

War crimes are not isolated acts; they are patterns of persistent and widespread violations of international law that are directed, authorized, or ignored by government officials. It is usually impossible to trace responsibility for an individual atrocity up the chain of command. One cannot find Slobodan Milošević's warrant for each atrocity in Bosnia. Bottom-to-top investigations of responsibility for war crimes disappear into a mist of battalion-, regiment-, brigade-, or division-level policies, practices, and understandings.

War crimes need not inflict civic destruction of the magnitude perpetrated by a Hitler or a Stalin. There is no minimum body count, such as fifty thousand murders, that qualifies Uganda's Idi Amin, Serbia's Milošević, or Guatemala's José Efraín Ríos Montt for indictment but exempts Chile's Augusto Pinochet or the Argentine junta of Jorge Rafael Videla. Even so, Amnesty International's secretary general was mistakenly hyperbolic in calling Guantánamo Bay "the Gulag of our times."[46] The Russian acronym GULAG, for "Main Directorate of Corrective Labor Camps," entered colloquial English from Aleksandr Solzhenitsyn's *The Gulag Archipelago*, which described Stalin's massive system of arbitrary arrest, secret trials, abuse, and inaccessible prisons. By any measure, Stalin's gulag dwarfs the prisons of the U.S. war on terror. The U.S. prisons are not a gulag, but they are an administratively coherent archipelago of facilities stretching around the world.

Unlike the people in Stalin's Soviet Union, no U.S. official risked disappearing into the prisons for dissent. Senior State Department and Defense Department officials, field commanders, intelligence and FBI officers, and frontline soldiers dissented. They were usually ignored. A few were threatened with administrative sanctions; a few were reassigned; a few requested reassignment. The possibility of dissent makes the silence and complicity of senior and frontline medical personnel in the abuse and neglect of prisoners that much more inexplicable and inexcusable.

The Geneva Conventions define the laws of wartime imprisonment. They also define war crimes. "Grave breaches" of the conventions are those involving any of the following acts, if committed against persons or property protected by the Convention: willful killing, torture or inhuman treatment, . . . willfully causing great suffering or serious injury to body or health.

In the preceding chapters, I have described violations of medical ethics and the Geneva Conventions pertaining to medical care and medical personnel. Some of these violations allowed "killing, torture or inhuman treatment" or "great suffering or serious injury to body or health" to proceed. Senior and frontline medical personnel assisted in or allowed three such breaches.

First, they allowed and assisted harsh and coercive interrogations. They cleared prisoners for these interrogations and monitored interrogations in progress. In this latter capacity, they had the authority to terminate the interrogations (and thus tacitly allowed such interrogations to continue). They applied medical skills and used clinical information about individual prisoners for nontherapeutic purposes.

Second, they failed to ensure that findings pertaining to the cause of death were reliably, truthfully, and promptly communicated to a prisoner-of-war information bureau to be made available to families and to parties endeavoring to prevent the abuse of prisoners. These failures contributed to an environment that endangered other prisoners.

Third, they failed to forcefully advocate for minimally adequate resources to meet prisoners' basic needs for mental health care, sanitation, tuberculosis treatment, shelter from weapon fire, and in some cases medical care. "Ghost prisoners" were at particular risk of neglect and abuse.

This list is confined to military medicine. It does not address, for example, the practice of sending prisoners to other countries for brutal interrogation, although I believe that the United States has an ongoing responsibility for such persons' well-being. It does not address the culpability of President Bush. His directive suspending the Geneva Conventions was a foundation for prison health violations, but his only order concerning the prison medical system directs that prisoners be "afforded adequate food, drinking water, shelter, clothing and medical treatment."[47]

My opinions about these breaches are those of a medical expert witness and not an expert in international law. A medical expert attests to the "merit" of a case. I have described my qualifications and listed authoritative standards of medical care. I have identified the records and facts that I have relied on. I have discussed the harms that resulted from failing to conform to those standards. A medical expert offers a professional opinion of whether a clinician has committed malpractice. An expert may also express an opinion of whether the executives of a health care institution negligently failed to provide adequate equipment, staffing, policies, and training for proper health care. In my opinion, "this case has merit"; it is up to lawyers, judges, or history to render verdicts.

THE GRAVITY OF THE CRIMES

After World War II, a horrified international community created standards to protect prisoners. In so doing, it rejected the idea that national sovereignty or the constitutional power of any chief executive encompassed a right to abuse, neglect, or torture prisoners. The signatories could not agree on how to police those commitments, so they elected moral suasion.[48] Thus, the international antitorture documents are unilateral promises to forswear cruel treatment, torture, outrages upon personal dignity, and humiliating and degrading treatment "at any time and in any place." In this respect, they differ from trade agreements, in which a violation by one party may authorize another party to respond with import duties or export subsidies that are otherwise barred. In signing the antitorture commitments, the United States helped forge a global civil society. In secretly abrogating the same commitments, the United States has undermined that community and the legitimacy of its claim to lead.

It is easy to minimize violations of antitorture conventions. Such documents are usually written by elite committees rather than by democratically elected parliaments. Transgressors are rarely prosecuted. As Stalin famously retorted when asked to stop persecuting Catholics, "The Pope? How many divisions has he got?" Some critics argue that the very idea of universal human rights is indefensible because each culture and time has its own values. As the future U.S. attorney general Alberto Gonzales put it in a memo leading up to the president's order to annul our commitment to the conventions, "In my judgment, this new paradigm [the war on terrorism] renders obsolete Geneva's strict limitations on questioning of enemy prisoners and renders quaint some of its provisions."[49]

The drafters of the Universal Declaration of Human Rights anticipated the critique of cultural relativism. They came from Asia, the Middle East, Europe, and the Western Hemisphere. They commissioned an international survey of values to ground their work.[50] The declaration was affirmed by the UN General Assembly; only the Soviet bloc, apartheid South Africa, and Saudi Arabia abstained. The declaration has stood the test of time; its values are how we measure any nation's claim to be a civil society. Its statement "No one shall be subjected to torture or to cruel, inhuman or degrading treatment or punishment" is a truth that the world's moral community holds to be self-evident.[51]

To call the prisoner abuses war crimes speaks to the gravity of the offenses but does not define the nature of the harm. The harm extends beyond the bruises and deaths of prisoners and beyond their families' personal losses. In Iraq, the Abu Ghraib photos were followed by an immense drop in support for the American effort.[52] Historians will assess whether the abuses and that shift in public opinion fostered recruitment into paramilitary forces against the effort to stabilize Iraq. As Secretary Rumsfeld's advisers and the FBI predicted, evidence obtained by coercive interrogation or torture is difficult to use in trial.[53,54] The reputation of the U.S. armed forces has been tarnished. The psychological damage to the soldiers who abused prisoners remains to be assessed. Those traumatized veterans will have medical needs.

As Secretary of State General Colin Powell predicted, the United States lost credibility as a human rights advocate. In 2005, for example, the United States criticized China for extrajudicial killings, torture and mistreatment of prisoners, deaths in custody, coerced confessions, arbitrary arrest, incommunicado detention, and a lack of due process.[55]

China's prime minister replied dismissively: "No country should exclude itself from the international human rights development process . . . and give orders to the others." The Russian Foreign Ministry concurred: "Characteristically off-screen is the ambiguous record of the United States itself. . . . Double standards are a characteristic of the American approach."[56]

Secure in its faith in American exceptionalism, the United States saw no urgency about joining the world community to buttress international laws against torture. By acquiescing in the executive renunciation of the Geneva Conventions, Congress abetted the shattering of the authority of human rights benchmarks. Together, the president and Congress abandoned a fragile set of international norms that fostered civil societies, protected democratic voices in totalitarian states, and constituted a court of appeal for our endangered citizens who have been captured by violent regimes. We did not offer an alternative. Now we must rebuild, with truth, transparency, and reform.

TRUTH

It is a reasonable question: why speak of war crimes when there is no chance of trial or formal censure?

There is a reasonable answer: naming the officials and policies is a necessary step in reaffirming the legitimacy of international law and highlighting the need to strengthen it.

Within the United States, there is little enthusiasm for truth and accountability. The Defense Department has confined reprimands and trials to low-ranking personnel. The federal government has rejected calls to empower a special prosecutor or independent investigatory commission. State medical and nursing boards do not impose licensing sanctions for "legal" military activities. U.S. medical societies, for example the AMA, have no leverage other than moral suasion over members.

There is mounting dissent from the international community regarding the United States' human rights practices in the war on terror. A UN working group has concluded that the conditions of detention, the renditions of certain prisoners to other countries, the failure to impartially investigate allegations of torture, the prolonged solitary confinement, and the harsh interrogation techniques amount to inhuman and degrading treatment that violates the UN Convention Against Torture and the International Covenant on Civil and Political Rights. The UN group says that the Defense Department medical program is not operating in a manner consistent with the UN's Principles of Medical Ethics.

The parliament of the Council of Europe has concluded that many prisoners at Guantánamo Bay are being illegally detained and subjected to torture and cruel, inhuman, or degrading treatment occurring as a result of official U.S. policy.[57] That parliament also condemned "extraordinary rendition," the practice of transporting people to third countries for imprisonment and torture. Italy has issued arrest warrants for CIA personnel involved in secret rendition. Spain, Norway, Sweden, Portugal, and Switzerland are conducting similar investigations. The United Nations Committee Against Torture (CAT) ruled that Sweden violated international law by allowing the United States to send Ahmed Agiza to Egypt, where he was tortured.

As then–Secretary of State Colin Powell predicted, U.S. officials face possible legal actions. A German prosecutor deliberated two months before rejecting a request to investigate Secretary of Defense Rumsfeld, saying that the matter belonged in U.S. courts.[58] However, while that petition was pending, the secretary canceled a planned state visit to Germany.[59] Fearing prosecution of U.S. officials, the United States pressured Belgium into changing its war crimes law.[60] There will be other attempts to subpoena or indict senior U.S. officials, although it is unlikely that a war crimes trial will convene. In the short run, these efforts may limit the ability of subpoenaed or indicted officials to freely travel after retirement from official duty. The reputation of the United States will suffer for a very long time.

REFORM

Reform requires transparency. Secrecy allowed the abuses to fester. Three kinds of transparency are required.

The prisons must be opened. The names and locations of many prisons are concealed; they must be disclosed. The prisoners' names are not listed in a manner that conforms to international law; they must be listed. Prison doors are locked to private visits between human rights monitors and prisoners; the doors must be unlocked. Rendition for clandestine imprisonment in third countries must stop.

The investigations must be opened. Classified material that does not bear on national security must be declassified. An independent investigation to review and declassify government documents must be empowered.

The reform process must be opened. The Taguba, Church, Fay, Army Inspector General, Jones, and Army Surgeon General investigations all have proposed salutary reforms. The Defense Department revised its Guantánamo medical records confidentiality policy to bar clinicians from "actively solicit[ing] information from detainees for purposes other than health care purposes."[61] However, that policy continues to allow medical records to be reviewed for "any lawful . . . intelligence or national security related activity."[62] The Army Surgeon General rejected his investigator's recommendation that "psychiatrists and physicians not be used as members of a Behavioral Science Consultation Team (BSCT)."[63] Civilians from the legal, academic, human rights, and medical communities must participate in designing and monitoring reforms. Their participation will also create more informed experts to monitor and advise the government in the future.

CHAPTER 8

WHY OPPOSE TORTURE?

I AM NOT A SECRETIVE WRITER. WHILE WRITING THIS BOOK, I TALKED with friends, relatives, colleagues, and reporters. I corresponded with strangers who contacted me by e-mail, letter, and telephone. Many people, including a jazz club owner, the clerk who renewed my driver's license, and a barista, recognized me from press accounts of this project. They often approached with serious questions. Most were supportive; I received cards and even a jar of homemade honey. Some people asked why I immersed myself in such unpleasantness or how the research was affecting me. Some were hostile. I corresponded with them all. I referred those who asked how they could help stop the abuses to Human Rights Watch, the Minneapolis Center for Victims of Torture, the American Civil Liberties Union, and Physicians for Human Rights.

Two features of these conversations stood out. People on all sides of the issue were struggling with a question: how do these abuses comport with what the United States stands for? It was clear that Americans know little about the reality of torture. Although we are steeped in fictional torture, we are unfamiliar with how widely real torture is used, with its techniques, or with its effects on individuals and their societies. Fictional torture is usually depicted as taking place in enemy or alien poor countries. Many people are only dimly aware of the United States' disastrous complicity with torturing regimes in El Salvador, Batista's Cuba, Chile, Iran, South Vietnam, Guatemala, Argentina, Saddam Hussein's Iraq, or Shah Reza Pahlavi's Iran. Some people are so deeply estranged from the reality of torture that they simply denied that any torture could have occurred in Iraq, in Afghanistan, or at Guantánamo Bay. This distorted geography of torture went with a belief that the United States practices "torture lite" or that it must use a little torture lest it tie its own hands behind its back and thus fail to survive in a world of evildoers.

Many people expressed concern that writing this book endangered my life. Those comments reveal a disturbing fear of the kind of society that we are becoming. I believe that they implicitly reveal how official violence against prisoners is damaging American civil society. Such fear fosters the silence in which torture thrives and democracy withers. The implication that I, a citizen of the United States, should acquiesce to that fear also strikes me as deeply disrespectful to my colleagues in Turkey, Egypt, Chile, South Africa, Cuba, and the former Soviet Union who have assumed much greater risks to fight torture in their nations. Some of those colleagues have been jailed and tortured; some have had their children murdered. It takes little more than the courage to be inconvenienced to speak against torture in the United States. If we are at risk of worse, then it is even more necessary that we speak out.

Often, after I had spoken on the topic of this book, an audience member would rise and ask, with deep feeling, "What could possibly make a person capable of doing such things?" The scrubbed, smiling face of a youthful soldier giving a thumbs-up over a prisoner's battered corpse cries out for psychological analysis. Was she emotionally deprived or was she a victim of severe corporal punishment during her upbringing? As a child, did she torture animals? Were her parents bigots? Did the Army program her to sadism? No characteristic antecedent or personality type has been identified in those who torture. Torturers defy pop psychology and psychological autopsies.

Robert Jay Lifton's concept of "atrocity-producing situations" helps reframe these listeners' question. He coined that term while studying veterans of the war in Vietnam who were suffering as a result of participating in atrocities.[1] Dr. Lifton, a psychiatrist, wrote that atrocity-producing situations arise at the confluence of extreme stress, a dehumanized enemy, and the assurance that ordinary limits on conduct do not apply. He quotes a combat medic in Vietnam: "I delighted in the destruction and yet was a healer."[2] That medic's words strikingly resemble those of a medic who beat prisoners during his service in Iraq: "You get a burning in your stomach, a rush, a feeling of hot lead running through your veins and you get a sense of power. . . . Imagine wearing point-blank body armor, an M-16 and all the power in the world and the authority of God. That power is very attractive."[3] Dr. Lifton wrote that governments create atrocity-producing situations by using propaganda to dehumanize the enemy and deploying soldiers on dangerous and ambiguous missions to win the hearts of people whom they do not understand. Dr. Lifton's analysis of the social psychogenesis of atrocities is powerful—and it is natural to let his words direct our attention to the battlefield and the event.

Instead, we should follow Dr. Lifton's insight away from the soldier's atrocity to his or her society. Why was torture reborn after being rejected as barbaric and ineffective two centuries ago? Why do modern nations create policies and institutions that promote torture? The historian Malise Ruthven notes a difference between the purposes of torture (punishment, interrogation, etc.) and its social function.[4] The ostensible purposes of torture are rationalizations used by a society that has decided that torture is morally permissible and politically desirable. Torturing societies create mirrored netherworlds. As Vice President Dick Cheney put it, "We also have to work . . . sort of the dark side."[5] Torturing nations define an enemy by race, pseudo-race, or creed. The enemy is heretical and never of the true faith. The enemy is so radically different from patriots, orthodox believers, or decent citizens as to constitute a special class of humans who deserve torture even though innocents will be abused along with the guilty. The enemy is omnipresent; nearly invisible; organized into cells, fifth columns, conspiracies, movements. The enemy's irrational anarchists are armed with ticking bombs. Depictions of dirty and groveling torture victims show people who seem to be beneath and apart from humanity; such images themselves dehumanize the victim. Secret and special state organs and policies must be mobilized to fight this secret and special enemy.

A person sent me this e-mail in response to an article I wrote about prisoners in Iraq and Afghanistan who were tortured to death:

> who gives a dam about these sub human animals. You so called educated asses need to worry more about us americans and america which

is your country yes. so smarten up and care about us before you go off worrying so much about terrorists. Who by the way may or may not have been abused.

The anonymous writer accepts torture as vengeance. The thirst for revenge occasioned many e-mails. The following anonymous e-mail came after I published a paper on homicides by torture:

> [You show] nothing but sympathy for a group of merciless monsters who would kill men, women and children in the name of Allah without the slightest hesitation. Try listening to a tape of a man screaming for his life while his head is being slowly cut from his shoulders, while a bunch of Muslims are dancing and singing praises. See how well you take that.

Many people wrote that beheadings in Iraq explained or excused the brutality at Abu Ghraib. Television carried the Abu Ghraib photographs on April 29, 2004. The first of the eleven beheadings in Iraq occurred twelve days later.

Violent international extremists do threaten civil society. The attacks in New York, Washington, D.C., Madrid, London, Nairobi, Yemen, Egypt, Israel, Istanbul, and Bali merit a vigorous, internationally coordinated police action such as has been used against other international criminal organizations—for example, the Mafia and the Medellín cartel. However, I do not believe that the cause of such police work is advanced by demonizing the criminals to the degree that our transmogrified image of them leads us to mire our military and intelligence resources in Iraq and Afghanistan. Nor is it advanced by damaging our reputation and strategic interests through wantonly forsaking our advocacy of international standards for civil society.

Pursuing justice differs from being consumed by revenge. The former proceeds from crime to investigation, to trial, to punishment, and then to closure. Vengeance is a whirlwind, where atrocity justifies revenge, and revenge becomes an atrocity. Abraham Lincoln understood the danger when the cause of a just war was eclipsed by the wish for revenge:

Thought is forced from old channels into confusion. Deception breeds and thrives. Confidence dies and universal suspicion reigns. Each man feels an impulse to kill his neighbor lest he be first killed by him. Revenge and retaliation follow. And all this, as before said, may be among honest men only. But this is not all. Every foul bird comes abroad and every dirty reptile rises up. These add crime to confusion. Strong measures, deemed indispensable but harsh at best, such men make worse by mal-administration.[6]

Shifting the question from "What makes a person torture?" to "What is the societal function of torture?" transforms the problem. Although it is easy to see torture as a soldier's deed, more fundamentally it represents the culmination of a national commitment to write policies, raise buildings, and recruit staff to perform and protect the crimes. Torture arises in societies that are blighted by the politics of extreme dehumanization. In this view, there is nothing novel in how the United States became a torturing society. The government posited a mysterious, omnipresent, Orientalist enemy that was vaguely described as (pick one) Wahhabi, or Arab, or Muslim, or a personality cult of Osama bin Laden organized by an Al Qaeda–centralized or affiliate-decentralized or cell-structured or multicentric coalition: et cetera. Government lawyers devised new categories— "illegal combatants"; the "failed state"—to rationalize the plan to suspend international codes of conduct. The president issued a directive (1) suspending humanitarian law and (2) directing the armed forces to treat detainees "humanely . . . to the extent appropriate and consistent with military necessity."[7] Prisoners were rounded up and sent to secret prisons and before Kafkaesque tribunals. Red Cross monitors were locked out of prisons, given false information, and, especially, kept away from "ghost detainees." Hundreds of people were covertly transported to nations that imprisoned, interrogated, and tortured them on our behalf. Facts gave way to chatter. Charges based on evidence were supplanted by accusations based on secrets. A fitfully changing color of "alert" flickered throughout the land. High- and low-ranking officials were sheltered from accountability. Government inquiries into the scandal found that "Army doctrine" allowed but did not authorize or order torture over a two-year period while torture was rampant. Soldiers were regularly exonerated after perfunctory investigations, or were lightly penalized in hearings that concealed the crimes, the names of the victims, and the names of the accused. The loyalty of those who did not assent or join in the cry for blood was questioned. As President Bush said, "You're either with us or against us in the fight against terror."[8]

A torturing society must secure the passive assent or active complicity of its professions. For two years, rumors, hints, and complaints of torture floated through the society. During that pre–Abu Ghraib scandal time, intellectuals wrote essays lifting up anecdotes about France's successful use of interrogational torture in the war that it lost against Algerians whose animosity was fueled by that same brutality. Salon and barroom chatter bandied about the notions of "ticking time bombs" and of safety afforded by "torture warrants," while the inefficacy of interrogational torture, and torture's history of bursting through any levee built to contain it in licit channels, were rarely mentioned. The U.S. media focused on circus trials and contrived "reality television." In January 2004, a media and congressional frenzy exploded over the brief flash of a pop star's breast at a football game, while those same institutions ignored an Army press release about an investigation of human rights abuses at Abu Ghraib. Four months later, that investigation became public when the Abu Ghraib photographs were leaked to America and the country awoke with shock and awe. The modern netherworld of torture does not thrive in the light.

The humane and respected profession of medicine assented to the human rights abuses in the prisons. However, the complicity of various clinicians, senior medical officers, and civilian medical associations needs to be individually weighed. The vast majority of clinicians in military medicine are competent and caring professionals. They have been unjustly tarred by this scandal. Many civilian and military health professionals did not know of these abuses and thus bear no responsibility for actions by their colleagues. However, some senior military medical commanders, and the leadership of civilian medical associations, should have known and should have taken steps to know; ignorance can be culpable. The culpability of negligent ignorance is one matter; the culpability for actions in the face of abuses must be dissected with care.

The roles of physicians in Nazi Germany and the Soviet Union, compared with their roles in Brigadier General Jorge Videla's "dirty war" in Argentina and in General Pinochet's Chile, suggest an important qualitative dimension for evaluating medical culpability for human rights abuses in U.S. prisons in the war on terror. Nazi and Soviet physicians were architects of torture. Nazi physicians put their profession at the service of the party. They joined early and built a pseudoscientific foundation for anti-Semitism, called race hygiene. Physicians and politicians used that "science" to build and operate the machinery for Fascist eugenics, first killing the chronically ill, who were by definition genetic "defectives," and then, in the Holocaust, committing genocide against "inferior races."[9,10] Soviet physicians constructed a diagnosis of "sluggish schizophrenia" and put it at the service of the state for incarcerating and drugging political dissidents.[11,12] By contrast, the torture physicians of Argentina and Chile simply went to work in the prisons. They did what was asked of them and they did not report what they saw. The complicity and silence of U.S. clinicians, military medical commanders, and civilian medical societies are more like the behavior of physicians in this second category. There were enough clinicians who were willing to be culpably ignorant, silent, or actively complicit to staff the prisons and to allow the abuses to continue without medical challenge.

We now approach the question that titled this chapter: why oppose torture? Torture is easy to condemn and seemingly impossible to eradicate. Any society seems capable of resorting to it. It has been practiced by wealthy nations, such as Germany and France, and by poor countries, such as Liberia and Cambodia. It is practiced by nations that are officially atheist as well as by nations grounded in every one of the major faiths. It is a tool of dictatorships and of democracies. We do not understand its cause or prevention. We do not know how to abate it when it rages. Though sentiment against torture is widespread, few people devote much effort to this scourge. Perhaps "torture" is one of those civic problems whose time is not ripe, and would-be reformers should direct their efforts elsewhere.

We do know that torture does not advance long-term national interests. It does not procure reliable information; the lies that it elicits overload and confound intelligence analysts. Its evidence cannot be used in civilized trials. It alienates potential recruits and informants. It enrages populations at whom it is directed, and it mobilizes them against the government that practices it. It draws its practitioners into unworthy relationships with nations who torture their own peoples or who torture on behalf of others. It makes civilized allies less willing to cooperate with extradition and intelligence sharing. The experience with torture in the war on terror has not found a new value in torture; it has confirmed old lessons: torture is a fruitless, often counterproductive, use of state power.

Torture's effects on the torturing society are equally destructive. Societies mobilized to torture are weakened by the vicious dehumanization that they must propagate to support the practice. Torture laws erode respect for the justice of law itself. The honor and traditions of institutions like medicine, law, journalism, and the military are tarnished by acquiescence in torture. Political reputations are diminished when the false conceit that torture can be confined to narrow licit channels is discovered. Torture responds to the barbarity of terrorism in kind. Like the terrorism it would deter, torture undermines civil societies. The rejection of either must include the forswearing of both.

Although it seems that every society is capable of torture, it is also true that every torturing society produces people who resist the sirens of dehumanizing propaganda and the rationalizations for torture. They are beacons in despairing times: Raoul Wallenberg of Nazi Europe, Aleksandr Solzhenitsyn of the Soviet Union, and Aung San Suu Kyi of Burma. What led Dr. Michael Gelles, the chief psychologist of the Navy Criminal Investigative Service, to carry his protest of brutal interrogations at Guantánamo to the highest levels of the Pentagon? Sergeant Joseph Darby cited his Christian faith as the reason for slipping a disk with the Abu Ghraib photographs under the door to investigators.[13] It is not, however, that simple. Other soldiers invoked their faith as they used pain to force prisoners to denounce Allah. With Wallenberg's and Darby's names before us, the question "What could possibly make a person capable of doing such things?" is inverted one more time: why does every society that practices torture also create people who dare to oppose the practice? Again, there is no psychological profile of the upbringing or moral instruction of people who heed the call to keep civil society alive.

A study by the law professor Oona Hathaway of 160 nations suggests the importance of these voices. Hathaway found that a nation's endorsement of international laws against torture does not reduce the chance that it will resort to torture. However, she also found that when domestic institutions in such nations "use litigation, media exposure and political pressure" to expose violations of those commitments, those same nations move in the direction of compliance.[14] Civilian medical societies are a respected domestic constituency and part of an honored international community. They have a crucial responsibility in opposing torture. They have played key roles in challenging abuses in Chile, Turkey, the Soviet Union, and other nations. Governments fear that their antitorture advocacy will extend senior-level accountability. Hathaway's conclusion about the necessity of domestic antitorture advocacy seems to be holding true for the United States. The government has answered the public outcry against medical complicity in human rights abuses with four studies of military medicine.[15-18] With continued pressure, these studies can serve as a foundation for reform.

Clinicians are frontline monitors for human rights abuses in prisons. We are in prisons where the Red Cross never goes and we are there when it is not. We can discern physical and psychic injuries even if they are not disclosed and even if they were crafted to be indiscernible. Torturers need medical accomplices to keep prisoners alive as trauma is inflicted, to predict how severely detainees can be twisted, and to see that torture evaporates, leaving behind neither scars nor documentation. Medical complicity shows a prisoner that he or she is utterly beyond humane appeal; complicit clinicians inflict the torture of despair. Jacobo Timmerman, who was tortured during Argentina's Dirty War, put it this way: the doctor's "presence was terrible because he was the symbol that a scientific instrument is with you when you are tortured by the beasts."[19] The Holocaust survivor Elie Wiesel wrote of prison medicine in Iraq, "Am I naïve in believing that medicine is still a noble profession, upholding the highest ethical principles? For the ill, doctors still stand for life. And for us all, hope."[20]

It will require tenacious professionalism for medicine to remove the stain of complicity with torture in 130 countries where physicians and torturers work side by side. We might start by recalling the story of the birth of western medicine in ancient Greece. In grief over his beloved's death, Apollo, the god of healing and reason, dedicated their son, Asclepius, to healing. Asclepius ("Unceasingly gentle") married Epione ("Soothing").[21] Legend has it that the historical Hippocrates was a descendent of that lineage. Greek medicine of 2,500 years ago had two foundations. Medicine is a natural science: curses, sins, and prayers neither caused nor cured disease. Medical practice is a moral enterprise, grounded on the principles of justice and beneficence. The Hippocratic Oath speaks of those values in its vow to society, to patients, and even to the prisoners at Abu Ghraib,

I will use regimens for the benefit of the ill in accordance with my ability and my judgment, but from what is to their harm or injustice I will keep them.[22]

INTERROGATING GTMO 063:
CASE AND DISCUSSION GUIDE

Mohammed al-Qahtani was Guantánamo 063. A Saudi citizen, he allegedly was assigned by Al Qaeda to join one of the hijacking crews for the 9/11 attacks in the United States. He was arrested in Afghanistan in December 2001 and promptly sent to Guantánamo for extended interrogation. In 2008, charges against him were dropped "without prejudice," meaning that they could be reinstated later. It is widely believed that public reports of the abusive nature of this interrogation meant that he could not be tried. The prisoner claims that any admissions he made were only made to stop the mistreatment.

Four documents describe the interrogation. The first is an untitled eighty-three-page log covering a period from November 23, 2002, to January 11, 2003.[1] The log was released by *Time* magazine; the Defense Department admits its authenticity.[2,3] Its author is anonymous: "ORCON" [ORiginator CONtrolled]. The other documents are from an Army investigation initiated by FBI complaints about the interrogation.[4-6]

The interrogation of Guantánamo 063 can be looked at in several ways. First, it depicts a coercive interrogation and shows how medical and psychological personnel monitored the abuse. Second, it may reveal the conduct of a research project on a prisoner. Finally, the ensuing investigation shows how the Defense Department evaluated and essentially excused the abuse of prisoners. The first and second matters are most germane to this book. This case discussion guide has three parts.

- Part I shows how the medical staff monitored this interrogation and how they responded to medical complications arising from the abuse.

- Part II shows how the psychologists managed this interrogation and responded to the abuses.

- Part III considers whether the interrogation of Mohammed al-Qahtani was conducted according to a research protocol.

Each part contains numbered paragraphs of information. The data are followed by questions to start the discussion. At the end of this appendix, I give excerpts from international law and ethics codes to inform the discussion.

PART I: PHYSICIANS, NURSES, AND MEDICS

1. The log covers a period in the middle of al-Qahtani's interrogation that began earlier in 2002 and continued into at least 2003. For eleven days, beginning November 23, al-Qahtani was interrogated for twenty hours each day by interrogators working in shifts. He was kept awake with music, yelling, loud white noise, or brief opportunities to stand. Then he was subjected to eighty hours of nearly continuous interrogation before what was intended to be a twenty-four-hour "recuperation."

2. The first "recuperation" was entirely occupied by an emergency hospitalization for hypothermia that resulted from intentional chilling with an air conditioner.[7] Mohammed al-Qahtani's body temperature had dropped to 95 to 97 degrees Fahrenheit (35 to 36.1 degrees Celsius) and his heart rate had slowed to thirty-five beats per minute. While he was hospitalized, his body chemistries were corrected. An ultrasound was done to search for clots in his legs as a possible cause of edema; it was negative. The prisoner slept through most of the forty-two-hour hospitalization, after which he was hooded, shackled, put on a litter, and taken by ambulance to an interrogation room for twelve more days of interrogation that were punctuated by a few brief naps.

3. Al-Qahtani was then allowed to sleep for four hours before being interrogated for ten more days, except for naps of up to an hour. He was allowed twelve hours of sleep on January 1. For the next eleven days, the exhausted

and increasingly noncommunicative prisoner was allowed naps of one to four hours as he was interrogated. The log ends with a discharge for another "sleep period."

4. Clinicians regularly visited the interrogation cell to assess and treat the prisoner. Medics and a female "medical representative" checked vital signs several times per day, drew blood, and suggested enemas for constipation or intravenous fluids for dehydration. The prisoner's hands and feet became swollen as he was restrained in a chair. These were inspected and wrapped by medics and a physician. One entry describes a physician checking "for abrasions from sitting in the metal chair for long periods of time. The doctor said everything was good." Guards, medics, and a physician offered palliative medications such as aspirin to treat his swollen feet.

5. Intravenous fluids were regularly given over the prisoner's objection. For example, on November 24, the prisoner refused water; a captain-interrogator advised him that the medic "can administer IV [*sic:* the log's contraction for intravenous fluids of an unspecified volume is used throughout this appendix] fluids once the Captain and the Doctor on duty are notified and agree to it." Nine hours later, after taking vital signs, medical personnel administered "two bags" of intravenous fluids. Later that day, a physician evaluated al-Qahtani in the interrogation room and told him that he could not refuse medications or intravenous fluids and that he would not be allowed to die.

6. The next day, interrogators told the prisoner that he would not be allowed to pray if he would not drink water. Neither a medic nor a physician could insert a standard catheter into the vein, so a physician inserted a "temporary shunt" to allow an intravenous infusion. The restrained prisoner asked to go the bathroom and was given a urinal instead. Thirty minutes later, he was given "three and one-half bags of IV" and he urinated twice in his pants. The next day, the physician came to the interrogation room and checked the restrained prisoner's swollen extremities and the shunt.

7. From December 12 to 14, al-Qahtani's weight went from 119 to 130 pounds (54 to 59 kilograms) after being given six IVs. On December 14, al-Qahtani's pulse was 42 beats per minute. A physician was consulted by phone and said that "operations" could continue since there had been no significant change. (Investigators noted a second episode of slow pulse in February 2003, after the period covered by the interrogation log.) Al-Qahtani re-

ceived three more IVs on December 15 and complained of costophrenic (that is, related to ribs and diaphragm) pain. A physician came to the interrogation cell, examined him, made a presumptive diagnosis of kidney stones, and instructed the prisoner to take fluids. The next day blood was drawn in the cell.

8. The Army investigation focused on whether the techniques were authorized by Defense Department policy. They found that the prolonged sleep deprivation was authorized. Cooling with an air conditioner was authorized "environmental manipulation." Notwithstanding bradycardia (slow pulse) requiring hospitalization, the investigators asserted, "There are no medical entries indicating the subject . . . ever experienced medical problems related to low body temperature." The Defense Department did not allow an admiral's investigation to review those hospital records.[8] Army investigators found no evidence that al-Qahtani was physically assaulted and pointed out that medical records did not find "medical conditions of note."

Discussion Questions

See excerpts from international law and medical ethics codes, at the end of this appendix, for references.

1. In your view, is any part of the medical aspects of this interrogation "torture" or "cruel, inhuman, and degrading treatment or punishment"?
2. Who was responsible for al-Qahtani's physical health?
3. Is there a difference between the responsibilities of the medical personnel who came to the interrogation room to take vital signs or treat edema and the responsibilities of those who treated al-Qahtani during his hospitalization for hypothermia?
4. Discuss the actions of the medical personnel in relation to the ethics codes.
5. Discuss the ways that diagnoses and patient assessments were made, for example in paragraph 7.
6. Discuss the ways that treatments, including intravenous fluids, were provided and monitored.
7. Are the ethics codes unreasonable for prisoners of war?
8. Should any of the clinicians who saw or knew of this interrogation have reported it? If the military command did not act on the complaint, should

information have been passed to a group like the International Committee of the Red Cross or Amnesty International?

9. Should any of the physicians or nurses or medics who assisted or knew of this interrogation be subjected to licensing or criminal or professional sanctions or censure?

PART II: PSYCHOLOGISTS

1. In October 2002, before the events covered by the log, a BSCT psychologist oversaw the use of Zeus, a military working dog, which was brought to the interrogation room to growl, bark, and bare his teeth at al-Qahtani. FBI agents objected to the use of dogs and withdrew. Army investigators concluded that use of the dog was properly authorized as a technique to "exploit individual phobias."

2. The psychologist who chaired the BSCT at Guantánamo was logged as present at the start of the interrogation on November 23. On November 27, he suggested putting the prisoner in a swivel chair to prevent him from fixing his eyes on one spot and thereby avoiding looking at the interrogators. On December 11, al-Qahtani asked to be allowed to sleep in a room other than the one in which he was being fed and interrogated. The log notes that "BSCT" advised the interrogators that the prisoner was simply trying to gain control and sympathy.

3. The interrogation plan repeatedly used the prisoner's religion. He was subjected to techniques called "Good Muslim," "Bad Muslim," "Judgment Day," "God's Mission," and "Muslim in America." He was called "unclean" and "Mo" (for Mohammed). He was lectured on the true meaning of the Koran, instruction that especially enraged him when done by female soldiers. He was not reliably told, despite his asking, when the interrogation was coinciding with Ramadan, a time when Muslims have special obligations. He was not reliably allowed to honor prayer times. The Koran was intentionally and disrespectfully placed on a television (placement deemed to be an authorized control measure) and a guard "unintentionally" squatted over it while harshly addressing the prisoner. Army investigators concluded that there was "no evidence that [al-Qahtani] . . . was subjected to humiliation intentionally directed at his religion."

4. Transgressions against Islamic and Arab mores of sexual modesty were employed. The prisoner was forced to wear photographs of "sexy females" and to study sets of such photographs to identify whether various pictures of bikini-clad women were of the same person or of different people. He was told that his mother and sister were whores. He was forced to wear a bra; a woman's thong was put on his head. He was dressed as a woman and compelled to dance with a male interrogator. He was told that he had homosexual tendencies and that other prisoners knew this. Although he was continuously monitored, interrogators repeatedly strip-searched him as a "control measure." On at least one occasion, he was forced to stand naked with women personnel present. Female interrogators seductively touched the prisoner under the authorized use of approaches called "Invasion of Personal Space" and "Futility." On one occasion, a female interrogator straddled the prisoner as he was held down on the floor.

5. Other degrading techniques were logged. His head and beard were shaved to show the dominance of the interrogators. He was made to stand for the U.S. anthem. His situation was compared unfavorably to that of banana rats in the camp. He was leashed (a detail omitted in the log but recorded by investigators) and made to "stay, come, and bark to elevate his social status up to a dog." He was told to bark like a happy dog at photographs of 9/11 victims and growl at pictures of terrorists. He was shown pictures of the attacks; photographs of victims were affixed to his body. The interrogators held an exorcism (and threatened another) to purge evil Jinns that the disoriented, sleep-deprived prisoner claimed were controlling his emotions. The interrogators quizzed him on passages from a book titled *What Makes a Terrorist and Why?*, which asserted that people joined terrorist groups for a sense of belonging and that terrorists must dehumanize their victims as a way to avoid feeling guilty about their crimes.

6. Al-Qahtani professes to be a broken man who gave false information under pressure.

Discussion Questions

See excerpts from international law and medical ethics codes, at the end of this appendix, for references.

1. Army investigators concluded that the cumulative effect of this "creative, aggressive, and persistent" interrogation was "degrading and abusive" but did not constitute "torture" or "inhumane" treatment, but they did not define distinctions between these words. In your view, are any of the psychological techniques used in this interrogation "torture" or "cruel, inhuman, and degrading treatment or punishment"?

2. Who was responsible for al-Qahtani's mental health?

3. Discuss the ethics of the actions of the BSCT personnel, who were psychologists.

4. Are the ethics codes unreasonable for prisons in time of war?

5. Should any of the psychologists who saw or knew of this interrogation have reported it? If the military command did not act on the complaint, should information have been passed to a group like the International Committee of the Red Cross or Amnesty International?

6. Should any of the psychologists who assisted or were silent about this interrogation be subjected to licensing or criminal or professional sanctions or censure?

7. Michael Gelles, PsyD, chief of the Navy Criminal Investigative Service, learned of the al-Qahtani interrogation. As a psychologist and seasoned interrogator, he was shocked. He filed a complaint, which was supported by his superiors, and took it to the White House. White House legal counsel eventually dismissed the complaint and ratified coercive interrogations.[9] Should Dr. Gelles have considered passing information he had to nongovernmental organizations like the International Committee of the Red Cross or Amnesty International? Should government policy provide whistle-blower protection if he passed information to such an organization?

8. Despite his objections to the al-Qahtani interrogation, Dr. Gelles supports the engagement of psychologists in interrogations. He writes,

Having worked with law enforcement, the intelligence community and correctional officers, I am very familiar with the structure and function of detention facilities. I am too aware of how easily aggression can get out of hand, and how the well intentioned can become carried away with emotion and perverse purpose and drift across boundaries, all of which may result in aggressive, violent and humiliating acts to detainees. We know that well trained professionals, clear guidelines, established procedures and scrupulous oversight serve to keep in check aggression and the tendency to over identify with a role and a method. Removing trained professional psychologists from these settings will impact the degree of oversight and inevitably increase the likelihood of abuse, thus having precisely the opposite effect of what occurred as a result of my involvement at Guantánamo Bay.[10]

Do you agree with Dr. Gelles? How would you define the proper and improper roles for behavioral scientists in interrogation?

PART III: WAS THE INTERROGATION OF 063 PART OF AN EXPERIMENT?

The introduction to this edition of *Oath Betrayed* outlined the history of CIA research on stress, hypnosis, and drugs for interrogation. I did not give that background in the first edition because I had no reason to believe that research had been conducted in the war on terror prisons. Circumstantial evidence is leading me to believe that abusive research may have been done at Guantánamo and that an investigation of this matter is needed.

The "interrogation log" of Mohammed al-Qahtani is an odd document. Why was it made? What is the point of meticulously recording the prisoner's tears and bathroom privileges, digressions on dinosaurs, and reactions to the interrogators' playing checkers if the primary interest is intelligence acquisition? The peculiar content and structure of this document makes sense if it is the log of research on coercive interrogation. This would account for why it focuses on the emotions and interactions of the prisoner, rather than on the questions that were asked and the information that was obtained. From the nature of prior CIA interrogation research and the log, it is possible to infer a design of the research project. As a research log, this log appears to be a chronological recording of clusters of stimuli (a stressor and a "Theme") and emotional and verbal responses.

The interrogators used "Approaches" and environmental incentives to psychologically stress the prisoner. The Approaches are derived from the Army Interrogation Field Manual.[11] They are techniques for creating an emotion (for example, helplessness, fear, shame, resentment, hope, or despair) within the prisoner. Environment incentives include "head breaks," naps, provision of toilet privileges, exercise, prayer time, noise, sleep deprivation, restraint, noise, ridicule, and the like. These techniques included the following:

Approaches

"Respect" [prisoner must respect interrogators in order to be respected]

"Right path" [interrogator instructs prisoner in correct Arabic/Islamic language/culture]

"Your mission" [What is God's mission for you?]

"Good Muslim" / "God's will" [How will you be a good Muslim?]

"Judgment Day" [How will you face it?]

"Invasion of personal space" [often female soldiers getting close to or touching male prisoner]

"You are a failure"

"Futility"

"Pride and ego down"

"I control all"

"Tell the truth"

"Direct" [questions]

"Rules for the day"

"[Your friends are] Already captured and talking"

An Approach was combined with a "Theme." Themes seem intended to prod the prisoner to respond in order to obtain privileges, cleanse himself of guilt, retaliate at friends who have betrayed him, and the like. The idea of interrogational "Themes" resembles prior CIA work with "projective" psychological tests that asked persons to reveal information in response to ambiguous stimuli. The Thematic Apperception Test (TAT), for example, was developed by Christina Morgan and Dr. Henry Murray. During World War II, Dr. Murray, who also had a long academic career, was a lieutenant colonel in the Office of Strategic Services (OSS). After the war, the OSS was closed and the CIA was created. Dr. Murray joined the CIA to work on agent assessment, a line of research that evolved into offender profiling.[12] In the TAT, a job applicant, prisoner, or a person with mental illness is shown a picture and invited to express how it makes them feel or what they see in it. The Guantánamo BSCT Themes are as follows:

Themes

"9/11" [Sometimes with video/pictures of victims]

"Circumstantial Evidence" [of guilt]

"Level of Guilt (and Sin) with Evidence" [sometimes by attaching pictures of hijackers or 9/11 victims to prisoner]

"Leniency" [if you confess]

"Manchester Manual" [refers to a captured Al Qaeda document; suggests that we know the training that you had to resist this interrogation]

"Global War on Terror"

"Al Qaeda Used/Destroyed/Raped Islam"

"Bad Muslim"

"Muslims in America" [by your association with Al Qaeda, you are inflaming attacks against Muslims in America]

"Al Qaeda Is Falling Apart and Talking"

"Saudi Government Has Abandoned Your Cause"

"Condemnation" [Islamic world condemns Bin Laden]

"Read Cards" [fortune-telling cards stating, for example, that all the innocent spirits will haunt him in this life and the next]

"Taliban" [are a debased sect of Islam]

"Attention to Detail" [prisoner is given irrelevant stimuli (e.g., pornography) or real-life details (e.g., his father's income), asked to recall detail and berated for inconsistencies]

"What We Know" [prisoner given facts and opportunity to reject them]

"Afghanistan"

"Justice"

"Rules Have Changed" [a rule for the interrogation is outlined and then abruptly changed]

"It Can Get a Lot Worse"

New Themes were being contrived and tested, as shown by the logged comment on the introduction of the "Right Path" Theme in the samples from interrogation logs given in the next paragraph.

Collectively, a Theme, an Approach, and an environmental incentive constitute a stimulus. Multimedia props were also used to complete a stimulus. These included videos such as "Taliban Bodies" or "Die Terrorist Die," fortune-telling cards, women's underwear, pornography, and so on. The log records two dimensions of response: the prisoner's emotional reaction (sadness, anger, silence) and content (relevant or tangential). The following are examples of how Themes, Approaches, and Responses were recorded.

SAMPLES OF COMBINATION THEMES, APPROACHES, AND RESPONSES

CIRCUMSTANTIAL EVIDENCE THEME

0425: Lead began session with "Circumstantial Evidence" Theme and "You are a Failure" Approach. . . .

0630: Control began session on "Circumstantial Evidence" Theme with "You have no Control" Approach. Detainee was attentive but unresponsive. . . .

0830: Lead and control started "Tell the Truth" Approach using "Circumstantial Evidence" Theme.

SAMPLES OF COMBINATION THEMES,
APPROACHES, AND RESPONSES

9/11 THEME

1225: Detainee offered food—ate one MRE and drank one bottle of water. Started "9/11" Theme. Detainee asked to pray when confronted with photos of child victims and was denied. Interrogators told detainee he was using religion as a tool to escape hard questions.

AL QAEDA FALLING APART THEME

0925: Lead starts "Failure" Approach with "Al Qaeda Falling Apart" Theme.

1000: Control puts detainee in swivel chair at MAJ L's [psychologist and chair of BSCT] suggestion to keep him awake and stop him from fixing his eyes on one spot in booth. Detainee struggled with MP when MP moved chair. Control used "onion" analogy to explain how detainee's control over his life is being stripped away. Control gives detainee three facts: we are hunting down Al Qaeda every day; we will not stop until they are captured or killed; we control every aspect of your life. Detainee did not speak but became very angry with control.

2030: Detainee was exercised for approximately fifteen minutes. The Medical Representative checked the detainee's blood pressure and weight. She cleared the detainee for further interrogation. Detainee refused water and food. Interrogation continued with the Theme of "Al Qaeda Falling Apart." The Approach that was used during this phase of the interrogation was "Pride and Ego Down" with an occasional "Fear Up" harsh if necessary.

RIGHT PATH THEME

1115: Interrogation team entered the booth. SGT B replaced SGT A. Team began the "Right Path" Approach with new Theme material written in English and Arabic. SGT B stated that he was now the detainee's teacher and should be respected as a teacher. Quotes from leading Islamic clerics that denounced the 9/11 attacks were read and shown to the detainee. Detainee was responsive.

The ritualized interrogation strategy seems designed to collect data and to develop a simple set of strategies to teach to inexperienced interrogators. It is unlikely that there is much substance to the Defense Department's claims as to the value or necessity of this coercive interrogation style. Secretary of Defense Rumsfeld referred to the Guantánamo prisoners as "the worst of the worst." Defense Department officials surmised that these prisoners had been trained on how to resist interrogation. From its point of view, such evil and well-prepared prisoners required enhanced "counterresistance" interrogation methods. The truth is more prosaic. Seasoned intelligence officers recognized quite early that a large majority of the prisoners at Abu Ghraib and Guantánamo had nothing to do with terrorism, insurgency, or Al Qaeda. The prisoners were indiscriminately picked up in sweeps or turned in for bounties. The few combatants had low rank and little information or insight. It is likely that brutal treatment made the prisoners less willing to talk. Four decades earlier the CIA's research program had concluded, "Interrogatees who are withholding but who feel qualms of guilt and a secret desire to yield are likely to become intractable if made to endure pain."[13] In the view of the National Defense University, that bit of intelligence has stood the test of time.[14]

In 1947, the judges at the Nazi doctors' trial created the Nuremberg Code in condemning Nazi doctors and health officials who were responsible for overseeing horrific experiments on prisoners.[15] From this foundation, research ethics, indeed modern medical ethics itself, was born.[16] Subjecting prisoners to abusive, harmful, and coerced experiments is a war crime.

Discussion Questions

See the excerpts from international law and medical ethics codes, printed at the end of this appendix, for reference.

1. Regardless of whether research was done in this instance, is the ban on coerced and harsh research on prisoners reasonable for prisoners of war?
2. If coerced and harmful research is found to have occurred at a U.S. military or intelligence facility, should collaborating medical, psychological, or behavioral science personnel be subject to licensing or criminal sanctions?

EXCERPTS FROM INTERNATIONAL LAW

United Nations Convention Against Torture

Definition of "Torture": any act by which severe pain or suffering, whether physical or mental, is intentionally inflicted on a person for such purposes as obtaining from him or a third person information or a confession, punishing him for an act he or a third person has committed or is suspected of having committed, or intimidating or coercing him or a third person, or for any reason based on discrimination of any kind, when such pain or suffering is inflicted by or at the instigation of or with the consent or acquiescence of a public official or other person acting in an official capacity. It does not include pain or suffering arising only from, inherent in or incidental to lawful sanctions.[17]

UNITED NATIONS BODY OF PRINCIPLES FOR THE PROTECTION OF ALL PERSONS UNDER ANY FORM OF DETENTION OR IMPRISONMENT

Definition of "Cruel, Inhuman and Degrading Treatment or Punishment": should be interpreted so as to extend the widest possible protection against abuses, whether physical or mental, including the holding of a detained or imprisoned person in conditions which deprive him, temporarily or permanently of the use of any of his natural senses, such as sight or hearing, or of his awareness of place and the passing of time.[18]

GENEVA CONVENTION RELATIVE TO THE TREATMENT OF PRISONERS OF WAR

In particular, no prisoner of war may be subjected to physical mutilation or to medical or scientific experiments of any kind which are not justified by the medical, dental or hospital treatment of the prisoner concerned and carried out in his interest.[19]

EXCERPTS FROM MEDICAL ETHICS CODES

UNITED NATIONS PRINCIPLES OF MEDICAL ETHICS RELEVANT TO THE PROTECTION OF PRISONERS AGAINST TORTURE

It is a gross contravention of medical ethics, . . . for health personnel, particularly physicians, to

[1] engage, actively or passively, in acts which constitute participation in, complicity in, incitement to or attempts to commit torture or other cruel, inhuman or degrading treatment or punishment, . . .

[2] be involved in any professional relationship with prisoners or detainees the purpose of which is not solely to evaluate, protect or improve their physical and mental health, . . .

[3] (a) apply their knowledge and skills in order to assist in the interrogation of prisoners . . . in a manner that may adversely affect the physical or mental health or condition of such prisoners . . . ; (b) certify, or to par-

ticipate in the certification of, the fitness of prisoners . . . for any form of treatment or punishment that may adversely affect their physical or mental health . . . or to participate in any way in the infliction of any such treatment or punishment . . . ,

[4] participate in any procedure for restraining a prisoner . . . unless such a procedure is determined in accordance with purely medical criteria as being necessary for the protection of the physical or mental health or the safety of the prisoner or detainee himself . . . and presents no hazard to his physical or mental health.[20]

WORLD MEDICAL ASSOCIATION

The doctor's fundamental role is to alleviate the distress of his or her fellow men, and no motive whether personal, collective or political shall prevail against this higher purpose.

For the purpose of this Declaration, torture is defined as the deliberate, systematic or wanton infliction of physical or mental suffering by one or more persons acting alone or on the orders of any authority, to force another person to yield information, to make a confession, or for any other reason.

The doctor shall not countenance, condone or participate in the practice of torture or other forms of cruel, inhuman or degrading procedures, whatever the offence of which the victim of such procedure is suspected, accused or guilty, and whatever the victim's belief or motives, and in all situations, including armed conflict and civil strife.

The doctor shall not provide any premises, instruments, substances or knowledge to facilitate the practice of torture or other forms of cruel, inhuman or degrading treatment or to diminish the ability of the victim to resist such treatment. The doctor shall not be present during any procedure during which torture or other forms of cruel, inhuman or degrading treatment are used or threatened.[21]

AMERICAN MEDICAL ASSOCIATION

Physicians must neither conduct nor directly participate in an interrogation, because a role as physician-interrogator undermines the physician's role as healer and thereby erodes trust in both the individual physician-interrogator and in the medical profession. Physicians should not monitor interrogations with the intention of intervening in the process, because this constitutes direct participation in interrogation. Physicians may participate in developing effective interrogation strategies that are not coercive but are humane and respect the rights of individuals. When physicians have reason to believe that interrogations are coercive, they must report their observations to the appropriate authorities. If authorities are aware of coercive interrogations but have not intervened, physicians are ethically obligated to report the offenses to independent authorities that have the power to investigate or adjudicate such allegations.[22]

AMERICAN PSYCHIATRIC ASSOCIATION

No psychiatrist should participate directly in the interrogation of persons held in custody. . . . Direct participation includes being present in the interrogation room, asking or suggesting questions, or advising authorities on the use of specific techniques of interrogation with particular detainees. However, psychiatrists may provide training to military or civilian investigative or law enforcement personnel on recognizing and responding to persons with mental illnesses, on the possible medical and psychological effects of particular techniques and conditions of interrogation, and on other areas within their professional expertise.[23]

ROYAL COLLEGE OF PSYCHIATRISTS

a. It is a gross contravention of medical ethics, as well as an offence under applicable international instruments and UK law for health personnel, particularly registered medical practitioners, to engage, actively or passively, in acts which constitute participation in, complicity in, incitement to or attempts to commit torture or other cruel, inhuman or degrading treatment or punishment.

b. Health personnel are only to be involved in professional relationships with prisoners or detainees for the purposes of evaluating, protecting or improving their physical and mental health.

c. Health personnel are not to: (i.) Apply their knowledge and skills in order to assist in the interrogation of prisoners and detainees in a manner that may adversely affect their physical or mental health; this includes certifying or stating that a detainee meets a specific mental or physical standard for interrogation. (ii.) Certify, or to participate in the certification of, the fitness of prisoners or detainees for any form of treatment or punishment that may adversely affect their physical or mental health, or to participate in any way in the infliction of any such treatment or punishment. (iii.) Question detainees about matters unless they are relevant to their medical care.[24]

Nuremberg Code

The voluntary consent of the human subject is absolutely essential. This means that the person involved should have legal capacity to give consent; should be so situated as to be able to exercise free power of choice, without the intervention of any element of force, fraud, deceit, duress, over-reaching, or other ulterior form of constraint or coercion; and should have sufficient knowledge and comprehension of the elements of the subject matter involved as to enable him to make an understanding and enlightened decision. This latter element requires that before the acceptance of an affirmative decision by the experimental subject there should be made known to him the nature, duration, and purpose of the experiment; the method and means by which it is to be conducted; all inconveniences and hazards reasonable to be expected; and the effects upon his health or person which may possibly come from his participation in the experiment.

The duty and responsibility for ascertaining the quality of the consent rests upon each individual who initiates, directs or engages in the experiment. It is a personal duty and responsibility which may not be delegated to another with impunity.

The experiment should be such as to yield fruitful results for the good of society, unprocurable by other methods or means of study, and not random and unnecessary in nature.

The experiment should be so designed and based on the results of animal experimentation and a knowledge of the natural history of the disease or other problem under study that the anticipated results will justify the performance of the experiment.

The experiment should be so conducted as to avoid all unnecessary physical and mental suffering and injury.

No experiment should be conducted where there is an a priori reason to believe that death or disabling injury will occur; except, perhaps, in those experiments where the experimental physicians also serve as subjects.

The degree of risk to be taken should never exceed that determined by the humanitarian importance of the problem to be solved by the experiment.

Proper preparations should be made and adequate facilities provided to protect the experimental subject against even remote possibilities of injury, disability, or death.

The experiment should be conducted only by scientifically qualified persons. The highest degree of skill and care should be required through all stages of the experiment of those who conduct or engage in the experiment.

During the course of the experiment the human subject should be at liberty to bring the experiment to an end if he has reached the physical or mental state where continuation of the experiment seems to him to be impossible.

During the course of the experiment the scientist in charge must be prepared to terminate the experiment at any stage, if he has probable cause to believe, in the exercise of the good faith, superior skill and careful judgment required of him, that a continuation of the experiment is likely to result in injury, disability, or death to the experimental subject.[25]

THE AMERICAN PSYCHOLOGICAL ASSOCIATION AND WAR ON TERROR INTERROGATIONS

Bradley Olson, PhD
Foley Center for the Study of Lives,
School of Education and Social Policy
Northwestern University

Steven H. Miles, MD

The American Psychological Association (APA) is unique among health professional associations in legitimizing U.S. interrogation policies and practices in the "war on terror" and particularly the U.S. government's claim that "we do not torture." Its collaboration with the Defense Department shows how a democratic society with decentralized authority uses scientific jargon and recruits diverse sectors to legitimize harsh policies. These sectors include law, the media, and professional societies. Such complex recruiting is not necessary in regimes with centralized power.

Many of the policies underlying clinicians' involvement with interrogations and Behavioral Science Consultation Teams (BSCT) were discussed in the introduction and chapters 3 and 7. This appendix elaborates on three less-covered topics. It examines why psychologists took techniques used to prepare U.S. soldiers to withstand captivity to use in the interrogations of prisoners in its own custody. Second, it examines the relationship between the Defense Department and the APA that led the APA to give its imprimatur to interrogations based on the inherently abusive paradigm of "learned help-lessness." Finally, it looks at the public reception of that relationship and endorsement.

The introduction sketched the long history of military interrogation research. Appendix 1 mentioned Dr. Henry A. Murray and his work with the CIA. The Defense Department also works with private psychology consultants and corporations. For example, Human Resources Resource Organization (HumRRO) was founded by the psychologist and APA officer Meredith Crawford, now deceased. It works on issues as diverse as recruitment of soldiers, interrogations, brainwashing, and training soldiers to be more likely to fire at an enemy. HumRRO personnel have held many APA leadership positions. The APA often calls on HumRRO personnel to give testimony for defense appropriations.

Thus, it is not surprising that defense and intelligence agencies turned to government and civilian psychologists during the war on terror. This time, however, business as usual produced a firestorm. There was an increased appreciation for human rights and disgust at the detention abuses at Guantánamo and the CIA blacksites. There was mistrust based on previous deceptions about prison conditions and how the U.S. administration had rejected international laws pertaining to the treatment of prisoners.

PSYCHOLOGISTS AS REVERSE ENGINEERS: BREAK THEM DOWN

Psychologist oversight of torture and cruel, inhuman, and degrading treatment for war on terror interrogations began in early 2002 in Afghanistan. Techniques from the SERE (Survival, Evasion, Resistance, Escape) program had long been used to prepare soldiers for harsh captivity. They migrated to interrogation policies. In March 2002, James Mitchell, a former SERE psychologist, cited Martin Seligman's experiments—shocking dogs to create "learned helplessness"—to advocate that Abu Zubaydah be treated "like a dog in a cage."[1] CIA psychologists, with Mitchell and Bruce Jessen, helped import SERE techniques to these brutal interrogations under the authorization of Secretary of State Rumsfeld at a secret CIA facility in Thailand.[2] Zubaydah gave up little information once abusive techniques were used.

Records from the Defense Department Office of Inspector General and the Senate Armed Services Committee (SASC) tell how SERE techniques were "reverse engineered" for harsh interrogation. SERE is a program to prepare U.S. soldiers to withstand captivity. Soldiers are abused as psychologists monitor their well-being. SERE techniques include restraint, heat, cold, isolation, sleep deprivation, desecrating the Bible, and even waterboarding. Although SERE techniques imitated communist techniques for getting "confessions," they have never been validated for effective interrogation. In July 2002, the Defense Department Office of General Counsel asked Lieutenant Colonel Daniel Baumgartner to obtain information regarding the value of SERE techniques for interrogations from resistant prisoners.[3] Baumgartner in turn contacted, among others, Dr. Jerald Ogrisseg, a SERE psychologist who was responsible for psychological aspects of SERE training. Baumgartner asked for details about the techniques and whether people were harmed by them. Dr. Ogrisseg told Baumgartner that SERE training was rarely harmful because it was monitored, the soldier undergoing the training or an instructor could stop it at any point, and the soldiers were assessed, debriefed, and, if necessary, treated for stress trauma.[4] Dr. Ogrisseg told Baumgartner that SERE techniques had never been validated for interrogation.

There is a critical difference between the risks of SERE techniques when used in a program designed to protect soldiers from acquiring a stress disorder during captivity and their risks when used to break a prisoner down for interrogation.[5] SERE trainees know that they will not be killed and that they can stop the abuse. Prisoners being interrogated have neither assurance. This lack of assurance is the centerpiece of the psychological theory behind war on terror interrogations: learned helplessness.

Learned helplessness came from an experiment conducted by the psychologist Martin Seligman. Seligman repeatedly shocked dogs that were held in a harness. He showed that the dogs could be conditioned to no longer try to escape the aversive situation, even when they were not being held down.[6] This experiment lies behind the SERE-based interrogations that aim to break the prisoner's will to resist the interrogator. On a cognitive human level, people who have some belief that they can control how they experience abuse are less likely to suffer stress disorders than people lacking this sense of efficacy to overcome the situational forces. SERE training, in essence, is designed to inculcate that belief of control in soldiers who are at risk of capture. When that belief is stripped away by counterresistance interrogation, learned helplessness ensues. Here, the risk of posttraumatic stress disorder is heightened. CIA research (see chapter 1) and a recent report by the National Intelligence Defense University (see introduction) have found that learned helplessness is an ineffective method of interrogation. Nevertheless, the Defense Department made expertise on learned helplessness a prerequisite for war on terror psychologists.[7] Thus, psychologically designed plans of torture and cruel, inhuman, and degrading treatment became U.S. policy. In May 2002, CIA and SERE asked Dr. Seligman to give them a three-hour briefing on the concept. When they turned discussion to its use in interrogation, however, he told them "since I was (and am) a civilian with no security clearance that they could not discuss American methods of interrogation with me."[8,9] Dr. Seligman denies further government contact on this matter.

Many of the steps, decisions, and commands by which SERE techniques were reverse-engineered to create interrogation strategies centered on learned helplessness remain unknown. It is clear, however, that psychologists were centrally involved at every step in crafting and implementing this interrogation model. In 2002, Colonel Morgan Banks, who was later appointed to the APA's interrogation policy task force, organized a meeting at Fort Bragg to apply SERE techniques to interrogation.[3] The agenda and attendees are not yet known. Later, he told the APA's interrogation policy task force that psychologists must be present during interrogations because SERE-based interrogators were in danger of going too far (so-called behavioral drift) "every five minutes."[10]

SERE psychologists trained BSCTs, which created interrogation plans to exploit prisoners' physical and emotional vulnerabilities. Psychologists and psychiatrists chaired these committees and wrote interrogation plans based on that training. (See introduction and chapter 3.) As the Defense Department built the system of cruel, inhuman, and degrading treatment that was required for interrogation by learned helplessness, it needed a legitimizing partner. If such a partner could sign off on rules for interrogation by learned helplessness, then ethical objections and perhaps even legal or professional sanctions could be deflected. A network of relationships between the interrogation rooms and the APA was built.

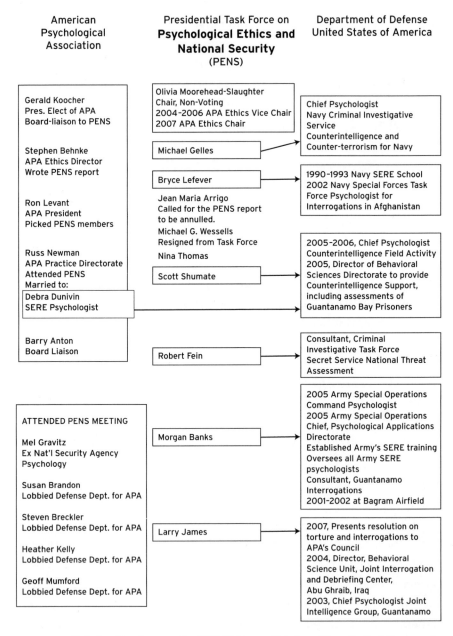

FIGURE A.1. *Relationships between the APA's Ethics and National Security Task Force and the Department of Defense. Used by permission of Trudy Bond.*

THE APA'S RULES FOR WAR ON TERROR INTERROGATIONS

From its inception, the APA's Psychological Ethics and National Security (PENS) Task Force was sure to be controversial. The members included a Who's Who of psychologist-interrogation experts who had held leadership roles in the problematic policies and facilities that the task force was supposed to address. It is not known how the APA selected these members or how this key task force came to be controlled by a bloc of defense and intelligence personnel. It is clear that the APA failed to manage the conflicts of interest. Defense Department members controlled content and access to the PENS deliberations. Assisted by APA officials and members, this majority sealed minutes and prevented public discussion of intermediate work products while they updated the Defense Department about the developing policy. Members' biographies are summarized in figure A.1.[11]

- Colonel Morgan Banks, PhD, is chief of the Psychological Applications Directorate of Army Special Operations Command. In 2001 he worked at Bagram in Afghanistan. He is the senior Army SERE psychologist. As noted earlier, he played a key role in organizing SERE education for the BSCT psychologists.[3]

- Dr. Scott Shumate was director of behavioral science for counterintelligence field activity for the Defense Department at Guantánamo. He had worked at the CIA's Counter Terrorist Center, where he supervised the SERE and learned helplessness–based interrogator-psychologists James Mitchell and Bruce Jessen. He reportedly left the blacksite where Abu Zubaydah was being interrogated under torture and eventually the CIA for the Defense Department because he disagreed with the harsh nature of Zubaydah's interrogation.[8]

- Lieutenant Colonel Larry James, PhD, served as chief psychologist for the Joint Intelligence Group at Guantánamo in 2003. In 2004, he directed the BSCT at Abu Ghraib during the postabuse period. During his first tour at Guantánamo, Lieutenant Colonel James would have been aware of or involved in standard procedures for Guantánamo that left detainees in isolation for thirty days to "soften them up" for interrogations and to create a greater psychological dependency on the interrogators. James claims in his book, *Fixing Hell*, that he heroically struggled to reform Abu Ghraib. However, when asked if he was aware of how high-value prisoners were treated in the most secret prison compound at Guantánamo, he said, "I learned a long, long time ago, if I'm going to be successful in the Intel [Intelligence] community, I'm meticulously—in a very, very dedicated way—going to stay in my lane. . . . So if I don't have a specific need to know about something, I don't want to know about it. I don't ask about it."[12]

• Captain Bryce Lefever, PhD, a Navy SERE and Special Forces psychologist, was assigned to Afghanistan in 2002 to teach interrogation techniques.

• Robert Fein, PhD, a forensic psychologist, has a long consulting history with the Directorate for Behavioral Sciences of the Department of Defense Counterintelligence Field Activity and other agencies.

• Michael Gelles, PsyD, was chief psychologist for the Naval Criminal Investigative Service, where he conducted psychological assessments of criminals and victims. Appendix 1 discusses how he called attention to abusive interrogations at Guantánamo.

Four members, including the nonvoting chair, were unaffiliated with the Defense Department or intelligence programs. Olivia Moorehead-Slaughter, PhD, is on the Massachusetts Licensing Board for Psychologists and was on the APA's Ethics Committee. Nina Thomas, PhD, has expertise in treating trauma victims. Dr. Michael Wessells is past president of the APA's Division of Peace Psychology. Dr. Jean Maria Arrigo is an academic expert on intelligence ethics. Drs. Wessells and Arrigo have renounced the PENS product.

In addition, there were persons who observed and sometimes influenced the PENS meetings. These are listed in figure A.1. Dr. Russ Newman, head of the APA Practice Directorate, was very influential. The civilian members were unaware that his wife, Lieutenant Colonel Debra Dunivin, PhD, was a former SERE psychologist.[13]

Not surprisingly, the initial PENS report conformed to government claims as to the propriety of the use of health professionals in interrogations. Ordinarily, a psychologist owes primary loyalty to the well-being of a patient. APA ethics director Dr. Stephen Behnke states that the PENS report "prohibits threatening or causing harm through physical injury or mental suffering, since threatening or causing such harm, if not rising to the level of torture, would constitute cruel, inhuman or degrading treatment."[14] He never engages the inherently abusive nature of interrogation by learned helplessness. As CIA attorney Jonathan Fredman told an interrogation planning meeting at Guantánamo, torture "is basically subject to perception. If the detainee dies, you are doing it wrong."[15] Dr. Behnke maintains that the American Psychiatric Association's rejection of a role for psychiatrists in interrogation is based on a misplaced "attention to a single principle—Do No Harm— [which] leads the psychiatrists to de-emphasize the role of protecting society."[14] The APA–Defense Department mantra was "safe, legal, and ethical for all participants."

- *Safe* was defined by White House lawyers, who distinguished generally unacceptable "torture" from acceptable "cruel, inhuman, and degrading treatment." Government policy said that a torturer had to "specifically intend" to cause pain "that would ordinarily be associated with a sufficiently serious physical condition or injury such as death, organ failure, or serious impairment of body functions." Although the administration revoked this definition for the Defense Department, the CIA definition, which applies to most of the prisoners in question, remains classified.

- *Legal* is a nebulous concept in secret off-shore prisons, where high-value prisoners are kept from human rights monitors and independent attorneys, and where the 2006 Military Commissions Act gives the president the unappealable "authority . . . to interpret the meaning and application of the Geneva Conventions."

- *Ethical for all participants* meant that psychologists did not have the ethical obligation of treatment. Psychologists were soldiers. As such, their duties fell within the ethics of war. The 2006–2008 Defense Department's BSCT policy puts it this way: "The [APA] Ethics Code pertains only to a psychologist's activities that are part of their scientific, educational or professional roles pertaining to the profession of psychology. The code does not therefore have purview over the psychologist's role as Soldier, civilian or contractor that is unrelated to the practice of psychology."[7]

The Defense Department and intelligence agency members of PENS did not simply affect the content of the PENS policy; they were an intelligence conduit to the Defense Department. Colonel Banks, Lieutenant Colonel James, and Lieutenant Colonel Dunivin kept Army Surgeon General Kevin Kiley apprised of details of the developing policy.[10] Thus, the PENS process was closed to APA members but transparent to the defense and intelligence agencies. As the report was about to be released, Defense Department members of the task force directed that the report be sent to the White House and Secretary of Defense Rumsfeld before it was presented to the APA membership or the media.[10]

THE BATTLE FOR THE APA

If the Defense Department hoped that the APA task force's report supporting psychologists' role in interrogations would end the debate, they were to be deeply disappointed. The Defense Department and CIA voting majority, the task force's lack of transparency, and the degree to which it conformed to the needs of government agencies with a recent track record of abusing prisoners made it a flash point. The blaze continues as of this writing in September 2008.

The Defense Department and its PENS members have continuously supported the besieged policy. In August 2007, for example, Lieutenant Colonel James spoke against a doomed moratorium that would have barred psychologists from working with war on terror interrogations. James told the audience and reporters, "If we remove psychologists from these facilities, people are going to die."[16] His statement essentially confirms the abusive nature of the learned helplessness interrogation system. After the American Psychiatric Association (see page 132) rejected the APA policy, Assistant Secretary of Defense for Health Affairs William Winkenwerder announced that the Defense Department would prefer psychologists to physicians for Behavioral Science Consultants.[17]

Initial resistance within American psychology came from within the APA's membership. Broader public debate led to spin-off groups of dissenting APA members. Approximately four hundred APA members have registered with a group called "Withhold APA Dues."[18] Former APA officers and honors awardees have published letters of resignation. It is not known how many

APA members have quietly resigned. Articles in academic journals have largely been critical of the APA position.[19-21] Dr. Jean Maria Arrigo, one of the two civilian PENS members, has created an archive of the PENS e-mails and notes.[10]

The APA has aggressively defended its policy in its own publications and in the press. It also responds to opponents' blogs. The APA's director of ethics, Dr. Stephen Behnke, unsuccessfully tried to enlist the support of torture survivor treatment programs. The APA has incrementally modified the initial PENS report in 2006, 2007, and 2008 but continues to affirm its core position that psychologists may help design and monitor the learned helplessness paradigm of interrogating prisoners who are deprived of due process, independent human rights monitors, access to attorneys, and habeas corpus.[22] It has made lists of prohibited interrogation techniques, but it has not addressed the abusive and infinite combinations of such techniques. It promised but failed to deliver a casebook training guide for psychologists who are involved in these interrogations. It has asked to research "the most effective means of eliciting information from a recalcitrant subject."[23] The Nuremberg Code and the Helsinki Accord forbid research on prisoners that does not serve the prisoners' interest and they would condemn the type of coercive research necessary to validate interrogation by learned helplessness.

The controversy has drawn in other nongovernmental organizations. Psychologists' associations have also rejected the APA positions.[24-29] Physicians for Human Rights, the American Civil Liberties Union, and torture survivor treatment centers are publicly advising the APA to back off from its position approving collaboration during coercive interrogation.[30]

Within the APA, opponents of PENS are pursuing two strategies. They have nominated Steven Reisner for APA president, running on a platform of ending psychologist collaboration with interrogations. Second, they have successfully urged the membership to pass a referendum that states that psychologists should not work for the chain of command at extralegal settings such as CIA blacksites and Guantánamo.[31] Rather, it says, psychologists should work independently for the prisoners, much as human rights attorneys or monitors with the International Committee of the Red Cross do. The Defense Department has aggressively inserted itself into the internal affairs of a civilian professional association with a press release urging APA members to reject the referendum.[32]

The APA presidential election will be decided by the time this book is released. The fundamental issue of the future of psychology's relationship to coercive interrogation in the United States will remain open for debate, however. In this broader and global context, the APA's position is critical. Even if a humane policy could be implemented within extralegal U.S. detention settings, such a policy would give the green light to far less savory totalitarian torturing nations to recruit psychologists into abusive interrogations around the world. A battle for the soul of the psychology profession is joined.

WHY?

Why would the APA ally itself with such questionable interrogation procedures? Why would it give a green light to psychologists' working in secret sites with prisoners deprived of legal rights, sequestered from human rights observers, under an interrogation model premised on coercion? It is tempting to proceed from these questions to look for organizational interests of the APA in allowing the important PENS task force to be so dominated by defense and intelligence personnel. Such questions are half of the issue.

A government has self-interests, too. Why would defense and intelligence agencies so aggressively seek to infiltrate and control a civilian health professional association in order to have a couple dozen pages issued under its auspices?

The combined set of questions, some about the APA's interests, others about the government's, point to a larger question. What is the social purpose of this kind of partnership in a democratic society that has resorted to creating secret prisons where human rights abuses are pervasive?

The APA says that its purpose is to assist psychologists who work in defense and intelligence programs and to provide guidelines to prevent "behavioral drift," by which psychologically uninformed interrogators might wander into abusing prisoners. Neither world history nor the "war on terror" experience supports this argument. Psychologists were intimately involved in the numerous abusive interrogations, including those of Abu Zubaydah and al-Qahtani Mohammed Jawad (a minor) at Guantánamo, and BSCT-approved interrogations in Iraq. Given the concerns about abusive interrogations that had generated the PENS task force, the APA could have selected a more balanced committee, included human rights experts, had a transparent process for engaging larger groups of stakeholders, and addressed the issue of sanctions for psychologists who collaborated with abusive interrogations. It took none of these steps. Moreover, the APA has obstructed formal complaints about its own members when evidence shows participation in abuse.

The APA has some tangible self-interests on the table. Alfred McCoy suggests that the APA's stance may be partly motivated by the desire to seek an ally in its quest for the right of psychologists to prescribe psychoactive medications as psychiatrists do.[33] Dr. Russ Newman, an active participant-observer of the PENS task force, is a strong advocate for prescription privileges for the APA Practice Directorate. His wife, Lieutenant Colonel Debra Dunivin, was among the first psychologists to obtain prescriptive authority through a Defense Department demonstration project. Newman and Dunivin worked closely with former APA president Patrick H. DeLeon to create and promote the Defense Department's prescriptive authority program and lobby at the state level for the Prescription Privileges Movement (RxP).[34] Beside prescriptive authority, the APA lobbies for and benefits from defense appropriations.[35] In 2008, it lobbied for funding for the Counterintelligence Field Activity (CIFA) and benefited from large appropriations for programs to train military psychologists.[36]

The government has an interest here that is no less real for being somewhat less tangible. A democratic government needs to legitimize policies and programs. For example, a broad buy-in by churches, community leaders, elected officials, and indeed the whole society was required to make civil rights happen. In this light, the APA, speaking for a broad part of the health care community, is an important legitimizing partner for government. If healers say that the interrogation methods are acceptable, guards are less likely to dissent; the public is more likely to assent. Psychologists, as healers, claim the respect and expertise to define "safe, legal, and ethical" interrogations. Their presence makes it appear as if referees or shortstops are available and that any harm from learned helplessness–based interrogations will be minor and passing. With 150,000 members, the APA is the standard-bearer for psychologists' code of ethics. It is a powerful legitimizing force.

So, in this partnership with government, the APA has more at stake than prescriptive authority or some additional program appropriations. If by entering into the PENS process it could successfully play a leadership role in legitimizing powerful new societal policies and institutions, its influence and the stature of its members would be enhanced.

Whatever its motivation, the APA's effort to enter into a government relationship to legitimize morally and legally flawed war on terror interrogations has reached an impasse. On one side is the APA leadership and the continued support of the Bush administration during its last months for maintaining abusive secret prisons and interrogations, which the world community, most health professional societies, and now a majority of Americans reject. PENS opponents have been able to get the APA to make a series of cosmetic changes in the PENS product. Most APA members, however, are not engaged. Governments that abuse prisoners rely on the tacit support of disengaged citizens. As the clock runs down on these prisons, history will judge whether the APA was on the side of protecting interrogatees or of legitimizing the evil use of a healing profession.

BIBLIOGRAPHY AND NOTES

THE PRIMARY SOURCES FOR THIS BOOK ARE GOVERNMENT INVESTIGATIONS, testimony, and memoranda.

Journal citations use the format of the 2005 International Committee of Medical Journal Editors' "Uniform Requirements for Manuscripts Submitted to Biomedical Journals: Writing and Editing for Biomedical Publication." This compact format is as follows: Last name Initials (up to three, then "et al."). Title of article. Name of Journal Year; Volume (issue number if needed for journals not continuously page numbered through volume):page numbers. For example: Doe J, Smith S. Torture related injuries. Pathology 1999; 112:156–62.

Citations to government investigations and policy memoranda have been greatly facilitated by the compilation *The Torture Papers: The Road to Abu Ghraib*, edited by Karen J. Greenberg and Joshua L. Dratel. Its pagination will be used whenever possible.

Army and Navy criminal investigations and e-mails have largely been obtained through the American Civil Liberties Union's Freedom of Information Act lawsuit and are posted on the ACLU's website, http://www.aclu.org/tortureFOIA. Citations to these documents pose significant bibliographic challenges. In declassifying the documents, government officials redacted the names of some authors, as well as some subject headings and dates. The documents are neither catalogued nor indexed. Most, but not all, bear pagination stamps of unknown origin. Some have multiple paginations. A variety of prefixes accompany most, but not all, of these page numbers. The most authoritative are listed here.

DODDOACID (Department of Defense Army Criminal Investigation Division)

DOD (Department of Defense)

MEDCOM (Medical Command)

Detainees (FBI interrogation notes)

The citation format is: Author or deponent, office, Title of document, date page.

Some government or media documents were only transiently posted on diverse websites. Accordingly, I have not cited the URLs from which documents were originally downloaded. Hard copies of cited material are available for a copying fee to interested researchers. Citation formats to heavily cited documents are described below.

REPEATEDLY CITED BOOKS

Books are cited in notes thus: Author(s) year (if needed), page.

British Medical Association. *Medicine Betrayed.* London: Zed Books, 1992.

Greenberg, Karen J (ed). *The Torture Debate in America.* New York: Cambridge University Press, 2006.

Greenberg, Karen J and Dratel, Joshua L (eds). *The Torture Papers: The Road to Abu Ghraib.* New York: Cambridge University Press, 2005.

Levinson, Sanford (ed). *Torture: A Collection.* New York: Oxford University Press, 2004.

Lifton, Robert Jay. *Home from the War.* New York: Other Press, 1973.

——. *Nazi Doctors: Medical Killing and the Psychology of Genocide.* New York: Basic Books, 1986.

Ruthven, Malise. *Torture: The Grand Conspiracy.* London: Weidenfeld and Nicolson, 1978, 25–31.

Saar, Erik and Novak, Viceca. *Inside the Wire.* New York: Penguin, 2005.

Stover, Eric and Nightingale, Elena. *The Breaking of Bodies and Minds.* Washington, DC: American Association for the Advancement of Science, 1985.

Yee, James. *For God and Country.* New York: Public Affairs Press, 2005.

REPEATEDLY CITED DOCUMENTS

When those documents are contained in Greenberg and Dratel's *Torture Papers*, the pagination in that readily available compilation is used. A reasonably stable Web address is given for other documents and those documents' internal pagination is used, if they are paginated.

Army Inspector General. Detainee Operations Inspections. Jul. 21, 2004. Cited as "Army Inspector General in Greenberg and Dratel, page."

Army Surgeon General. Final Report: Assessment of Detainee Medical Operations for OEF (Operation Enduring Freedom), GTMO (Guantánamo), and OIF (Operation Iraqi Freedom). Apr. 13, 2005. Posted at http://www.armymedicine.army.mil/news/detmedopsrprt/detmedopsrpt.pdf. Cited as "Surgeon General, page."

Church, Albert. Executive Summary (of untitled review of Department of Defense interrogation operations). Mar. 2005. http://www.defenselink.mil/news/Mar2005/d20050310exe.pdf. Cited as "Church, page."

Fay, George R. Investigation of the Abu Ghraib Detention Facility and 205th Military Intelligence Brigade. Aug. 2004. Cited as "Fay in Greenberg and Dratel, page."

International Committee of the Red Cross (ICRC). Report of the International Committee of the Red Cross on the Treatment by the Coalition Forces of Prisoners of War and Other Protected Persons by the Geneva Conventions in Iraq During Arrest, Internment, and Interrogation. Feb. 2004. ICRC. Cited as "ICRC in Greenberg and Dratel, page."

Jones, Anthony R. Investigation of the Abu Ghraib Prison and 205th Military Intelligence Brigade. Aug. 2004. Cited as "Jones in Greenberg and Dratel, page."

Miller, Geoffrey D. Assessment of DoD Counter-terrorism Interrogation and Detention Operations in Iraq. Sep. 2003. Cited as "Miller in Greenberg and Dratel, page."

Ryder, Donald J. Report on Detention and Corrections Operations in Iraq. Nov. 2003. Posted at Center for Public Integrity, http://www.publicintegrity.org/docs/abughraib/abu5.pdf. Cited as "Ryder, page."

Schlesinger, James. Final Report of the Independent Panel to Review DoD

Detention Operations. Aug. 2004. Cited as "Schlesinger in Greenberg and Dratel, page."

Taguba, Antonio. Article 15-6 Investigation of the 800th Military Police Brigade. Mar. 2004. Portions that appear in *Torture Papers* are cited as "Section Name [e.g., Executive Summary] in Greenberg and Dratel, page." Annexes to the Taguba report that are not reprinted in Greenberg and Dratel are cited as "Document title. Taguba Annex #: page (if paginated)" (e.g., Sworn Statement of John Doe. Jan. 16, 2004, Taguba Annex 52:2). The Center for Public Integrity's website contains the available Taguba annexes: http://www.publicintegrity.org/report.aspx?aid=417&sid=100.

Working Group on Arbitrary Detention. Situation of detainees at Guantánamo Bay. Economic and Social Council of the United Nations. E/CN.4/2006/120. Feb. 15, 2006. Cited as "Working Group, page."

INTERNATIONAL CONVENTIONS, UN RESOLUTIONS, AND SO ON

Conference on Security and Co-Operation in Europe, Final Act. Helsinki Aug. 1975, http://www.hri.org/docs/helsinki75.html.

Convention Against Torture and Other Cruel, Inhuman or Degrading Treatment or Punishment, United Nations, 1987, http://www.unhchr.ch/html/menu3/b/h_cat39.htm.

Geneva Convention Relative to the Treatment of Prisoners of War, 1949, http://www.unhchr.ch/html/menu3/b/91.htm.

Geneva Convention Relative to the Protection of Civilian Persons in Time of War, 1949, http://www.unhchr.ch/html/menu3/b/92.htm.

International Covenant on Civil and Political Rights, United Nations, 1976, http://www.unhchr.ch/html/menu3/b/a_ccpr.htm.

United Nations, Principles of Medical Ethics Relevant to the Role of Health Personnel, Particularly Physicians, in the Protection of Prisoners and Detainees Against Torture and Other Cruel, Inhuman or Degrading Treatment or Punishment, 1982, http://www.unhchr.ch/html/menu3/b/h_comp40.htm.

United Nations Standard Minimum Rules for the Treatment of Prisoners, 1955, http://www.unhchr.ch/html/menu3/b/h_comp34.htm.

Universal Declaration of Human Rights, 1948, http://www.unhchr.ch/udhr/index.htm.

U.S. FEDERAL LAWS

War Crimes Act, 18 U.S.C. Part I: 118:§2441, http://www4.law.cornell.edu/
uscode/html/uscode18/usc_sec_18_00002441----000-.html.

Torture: U.S.C. 18: Part I; 113C—Torture.

Torture Victims Relief Reauthorization Act of 2005, http://www.govtrack.us
/congress/bill.xpd?bill=h109-2017.

MEDICAL ETHICS STANDARDS

American College of Physicians. Relation of the Physician to Government.
http://www.acponline.org/ethics/ethicman5th.htm.

American Medical Association. E-2.067 Torture. http://www.ama-assn.org/
ama/pub/category/8421.html.

American Psychiatric Association and American Psychological Association.
Joint resolution against torture. http://www.psych.org/edu/other_res/lib
_archives/archives/198506.pdf.

American Psychological Association. Ethics Code. http://www.apa.org/ethics/
code2002.html.

Amnesty International. Declaration on the Role of Health Professionals in
the Exposure of Torture and Ill-Treatment, 1996. http://www1.umn.edu/
humanrts/instree/healthprofessionalrole.html.

International Council of Nurses. Nurses' Role in the Care of Prisoners and Detainees, International Council of Nurses. http://www.icn.ch/psdetainees
.htm.

———. Torture, Death Penalty and Participation by Nurses in Executions.
http://www.icn.ch/pstorture.htm.

Istanbul Protocol. The Manual on Effective Investigation and Documentation
of Torture and Other Cruel, Inhuman or Degrading Treatment or Punishment, 1999. http://www.phrusa.org/research/istanbul_protocol/ist_prot.pdf.

World Medical Association. Declaration of Geneva, 1948. http://www.cirp
.org/library/ethics/geneva/.

———. Declaration on Hunger Strikers (Declaration of Malta). http://web
.amnesty.org/pages/health-ethicswmahs-eng.

———. Guidelines for Medical Doctors Concerning Torture and Other
Cruel, Inhuman or Degrading Treatment or Punishment in Relation to

Detention and Imprisonment (Declaration of Tokyo), 1975. http://web
.amnesty.org/pages/health-ethicswmatokyo-eng.

———. Regulations in Time of Armed Conflict. http://web.amnesty.org/
pages/health-ethicsregs-eng.

———. Statement on the Licensing of Physicians Fleeing Prosecution
for Serious Criminal Offences. http://web.amnesty.org/pages/health
-ethicswmalicense-eng.

World Psychiatric Association. Declaration of Hawaii, 1977. http://www
.codex.uu.se/texts/hawaii.html.

———. Ethical Standards for Psychiatric Practice (Declaration of Madrid),
1996. http://www.wpanet.org/generalinfo/ethic1.html.

INTRODUCTION

1. Miles SH. A troubling silence from prison medics. Associated Press May 18, 2004.

2. Bloche MG. After Abu Ghraib; Physician, turn thyself in. New York Times Jun. 10, 2004.

3. Lifton RJ. Doctors and torture. New England Journal of Medicine 2004;351:415–16.

4. Miles SH. Abu Ghraib: Its legacy for military medicine. Lancet 2004;364:725–29.

5. Army Surgeon General [e-mail]. Docs and torture. Aug. 20, 2004, MEDCOM 407. http://www1.umn.edu/humanrts/OathBetrayed/Medcom%20387–585.pdf. (Accessed Oct. 18, 2008.)

6. Zabarenko D. Doctors aided prison abuse. Reuters Aug. 21, 2004.

7. Olson J. U archives unvarnished look at war detainees. Pioneer Press Apr. 25, 2007.

8. Beaver D. Legal Brief on Proposed Counter Resistance Strategies. Oct. 11, 2002. http://www1.umn.edu/humanrts/OathBetrayed/Beaver-Phifer-Rumsfeld%2010-11-02.pdf (p. 5 of pdf). (Accessed Oct. 13, 2008.)

9. Secretary of Defense. Counter-Resistance Techniques in the War on Terrorism. Apr. 16, 2003. http://www1.umn.edu/humanrts/OathBetrayed/Rumsfeld%204-16-03.pdf. (Accessed Oct. 18, 2008.)

10. Miller J. Assessment of DoD Counterterrorism Interrogation and Deten-

tion Operations in Iraq. http://www1.umn.edu/humanrts/OathBetrayed/Taguba%20Annex%2020.pdf. (Accessed Oct. 18, 2008.)

11. Joint Interrogation and Detention Center. Organization Chart. Jan. 23, 2004. http://www1.umn.edu/humanrts/OathBetrayed/Taguba%20Annex%2040.pdf (p. 18 of pdf). (Accessed Oct. 13, 2008.)

12. Bloche MG, Marks JH. When doctors go to war. New England Journal of Medicine 2004;352:3–6.

13. Army Surgeon General. Final Report: Assessment of Detainee Medical Operations for OEF, GTMO, and OIF. Apr. 13, 2005. http://www1.umn.edu/humanrts/OathBetrayed/Army%20Surgeon%20General%20Report.pdf. (Accessed Oct. 18, 2008.)

14. Department of Defense. Medical Program Support for Detainee Operations. Jun. 6, 2006. http://www.dtic.mil/whs/directives/corres/pdf/231008p.pdf. (Accessed Oct. 18, 2008.)

15. Bybee J. Standards of Conduct for Interrogation under 18 USC 2340–2340 A. Aug. 1, 2002, pp. 9–12. http://www.washingtonpost.com/wp-srv/politics/documents/cheney/torture_memo_aug2002.pdf. (Accessed Oct. 13, 2008.)

16. Working Group. Detainee Interrogations in the Global War on Terrorism. Apr. 4, 2003. http://www.dod.mil/pubs/foi/detainees/working_grp_report_detainee_interrogations.pdf. (Accessed Oct. 18, 2008.)

17. Yoo JC. Memo Regarding the Torture and Military Interrogation of Alien Unlawful Combatants Held Outside the United States (3/14/2003), pp. 41–44. http://www.aclu.org/pdfs/safefree/yoo_army_torture_memo.pdf. (Accessed Oct. 18, 2008.)

18. Surgeon General Army. Final Report: Assessment of Detainee Medical Operations for OEF, GTMO, and OIF. Apr. 13, 2005, p. 20:9. http://www1.umn.edu/humanrts/OathBetrayed/Army%20Surgeon%20General%20Report.pdf. (Accessed Oct. 18, 2008.)

19. Warrick J. Detainees allege being drugged, questioned. Washington Post Apr. 22, 2008.

20. U.S. Senate Armed Services Committee. The Origins of Aggressive Interrogation Techniques. [Multiple documents, multiple dates]. http://levin.senate.gov/newsroom/supporting/2008/Documents.SASC.061708.pdf (pp. 14–18 of pdf). (Accessed Oct. 18, 2008.)

21. Declassified MK-Ultra Files (undated). http://www.michael-robinett .com/declass/c000.htm. (Accessed Oct. 18, 2008.)

22. Richelson JT. Science, Technology and the CIA: A National Security Archive Electronic Briefing Book, 2001. http://www.gwu.edu/~nsarchiv/ NSAEBB/NSAEBB54/. (Accessed Oct. 18, 2008.)

23. Rejali D. *Torture and Democracy.* Princeton, NJ: Princeton University Press, 2008.

24. United States Senate Select Committee. Governmental Operations with Respect to Intelligence Activities, Book I: Foreign and Military Intelligence, 1976. http://www.aarclibrary.org/publib/church/reports/book1/ html/ChurchB1_0197a.htm. (Accessed Oct. 13, 2008.)

25. Marks JD. *The Search for the Manchurian Candidate: The CIA and Mind Control.* New York: W. W. Norton & Company, 1991.

26. Mayer J. The experiment. New Yorker Jul. 11, 2005. http://www .newyorker.com/archive/2005/07/11/050711fa_fact4. (Accessed Oct. 18, 2008.)

27. Department of Defense, Office of Inspector General. Review of DoD-Directed Investigations of Detainee Abuse. Aug. 25, 2006. http://www .dodig.osd.mil/fo/Foia/DetaineeAbuse.html. (Accessed Oct. 18, 2008.)

28. http://levin.senate.gov/newsroom/supporting/2008/Documents .SASC.061708.pdf.

29. Mayer J. *The Dark Side.* New York: Doubleday, 2008.

30. United Nations Economic and Social Council. Situation of detainees at Guantánamo Bay E/CN.4/2006/120. Feb 27, 2006. http://www1.umn.edu/ humanrts/OathBetrayed/United%20Nations%20Working%20Group .pdf. (Accessed Oct. 18, 2008.)

31. Citizens for Global Solutions. California becomes first state to ban torture. http://www.globalsolutions.org/blog/index.php/home/2008/10/06/ california_becomes_first_u_s_state_to_ba. (Accessed Oct. 18, 2008.)

32. American Psychiatric Association. Psychiatric participation in the interrogation of detainees. 2006. http://www.psych.org/Departments/EDU/ Library/APAOfficialDocumentsandRelated/PositionStatements/200601 .aspx. (Accessed Oct. 18, 2008.)

33. American Psychoanalytic Association. Torture. 2006. http://apsa.org/ ABOUTAPSAA/POSITIONSTATEMENTS/TORTURE/tabid/468/ Default.aspx. (Accessed Oct. 18, 2008.)

34. International Psychoanalytical Association. Statement on torture. 2007. http://internationalpsychoanalysis.net:80/2007/09/11/ipa-statement-on -torture-passed-in-berlin-on-july-2007/. (Accessed Oct. 18, 2008.)

35. Royal College of Psychiatrists. Resolution condemning psychiatric participation of detainees. 2006. http://www.rcpsych.ac.uk/pressparliament/ pressreleases2006/pr825.aspx. (Accessed Oct. 18, 2008.)

36. United Kingdom Council for Psychotherapy. UKCP Statement on Torture. 2007. http://www.psychotherapy.org.uk:80/iqs/sid.098429402789 29031509767/UKCP_Statement_on_Torture.html. (Accessed Oct. 18, 2008.)

37. AMA Council on Ethical and Judicial Affairs. Physician participation in interrogation (Opinion 4-I-06). 2006. http://www.ama-assn.org/ama1/ pub/upload/mm/475/cejo4i06.doc. (Accessed Nov. 9, 2007.)

38. World Medical Association. Resolution on the Responsibility of Physicians in the Documentation and Denunciation of Acts of Torture or Cruel or Inhuman or Degrading Treatment. 2007. http://www.wma .net/e/policy/t1.htm. (Accessed Oct. 18, 2008.)

39. Miles SH. Doctors' complicity with torture: It is time for sanctions. BMJ 2008;337:a1088.

40. Church A. Untitled Report for Secretary of Defense. Mar. 2005. http:// www.aclu.org/pdfs/safefree/church_353365_20080430.pdf. (Accessed Oct. 18, 2008.)

41. Joint Task Force, Guantanamo Bay. Camp Delta Standard Operating Procedures. Mar. 1, 2004. http://humanrights.ucdavis.edu/projects/the -guantanamo-testimonials-project/testimonies/testimonies-of-standard -operating-procedures/camp_delta_sop_2004.pdf. (Accessed Oct. 18, 2008.)

42. A Review of the FBI's Involvement in and Observations of Detainee Interrogations in Guantanamo Bay, Afghanistan, and Iraq. May 2008. http://graphics8.nytimes.com/packages/pdf/washington/20080521 _DETAIN_report.pdf. (Accessed Oct. 18, 2008.)

43. The Intelligence Science Board. Educing Information Interrogation: Science and Art. National Defense Intelligence University. 2006. http:// www1.umn.edu/humanrts/OathBetrayed/Intelligence%20Science %20Board%202006.pdf. (Accessed Oct. 18, 2008.)

44. Working Group, 12.

45. Gillers S. Legal ethics: A debate. In Greenberg, 236–40.

46. Bowker DW. Unwise counsel: The war on terrorism and criminal mistreatment of detainees in US custody. In Greenberg, 183–202.

47. Miles S, Marks L (eds). United States Military Medicine in War on Terror Prisons. Human Rights Library of the University of Minnesota, 2007. http://www1.umn.edu/humanrts/OathBetrayed/index.html. (Accessed Oct. 18, 2008.)

48. Miles SH. Human rights abuses, transparency, impunity and the Web. Torture 2007;17:216–21.

49. Pross C. Burnout, vicarious traumatization and its prevention. Torture 2006;16:1–9.

PART I: "WE ARE SELLING OUR SOULS FOR DROSS"

CHAPTER 1: TORTURE

1. Jordon S. Sworn testimony. Feb. 24, 2004, Taguba Annex 53:48–53.

2. Sivits JC. Sworn statement. Jan. 14, 2004, Taguba Annex 25/26.

3. Al-Sheikh AS. Sworn statement. Jan. 16, 2004, in Greenberg and Dratel, 522 (partial), entire statement in Taguba Annex 25/26.

4. Layton R. Sworn statement. Jan. 14, 2004, Taguba Annex 25/26.

5. Sivits JC. Sworn statement. Jan. 14, 2004, Taguba Annex 25/26.

6. Layton R. Sworn statement. Jan. 14, 2004, Taguba Annex 25/26.

7. Fay in Greenberg and Dratel, 1051.

8. Fay in Greenberg and Dratel, 1081, 1102, 1121–22.

9. [Name redacted, of 470th Military Intelligence Group]. Sworn statement. May 18, 2004, DOD 000340-46.

10. Surgeon General, 20-15.

11. [Name redacted]. CJTF-TFF-1: Memorandum for the Record of Interview. Jun. 29, 2004, DOD 000347.

12. Shakespeare W. *Henry VI, Part 2*. Act 2, Scene 1.

13. Coetzee JM. *Waiting for the Barbarians*. Penguin Books, New York, 1982, 5.

14. Arrigo JM. A utilitarian argument against torture interrogation of terrorists. Science & Engineering Ethics 2004;10:543–72.

15. Schlesinger in Greenberg and Dratel, 974–75.

16. Randall GR, Lutz L, Quiroga J, et al. Physical and psychiatric effects of torture: two medical studies. In Stover and Nightingale, 62–63.

17. Thomsen JL. The role of the pathologist in human rights abuses. Journal of Clinical Pathology 2000;53:569–72.

18. [Name redacted]. Sworn statement. Sep. 20, 2003, DODDOACID 000113-16.

19. US Army: 43rd Military Police Detachment, 10th Military Police Battalion. Criminal Investigation Division Report-Final-152-03-CID469-60212. Feb. 6, 2004, DODDOACID 000105-66.

20. Military Intelligence Slide Show. TTPs [Tactics, Techniques, and Procedures] & lessons learned. [Undated], Taguba Annex 40:0001781.

21. [Name redacted, of A Battalion, 4th Infantry]. Sworn statement. Sep. 27, 2003, DODDOACID 000119-16.

22. [Name redacted, of D Battalion, 104th Military Intelligence]. Sworn statement. Sep. 27, 2003, DODDOACID 000142-45.

23. [Name redacted, of 4th Infantry Division]. Sworn statement. Sep. 27, 2003, DODDOACID 000134-36.

24. US Army: 43rd Military Police Detachment, 10th Military Police Battalion. Criminal Investigation Division Report-Final-152-03-CID469-60212. Feb. 6, 2004, DODDOACID 000111.

25. [Name redacted, of 4th Infantry Division]. Sworn statement. Sep. 27, 2003, DODDOACID 000119-21.

26. Sontag D. How colonel risked his career by menacing detainee and lost. New York Times May 27, 2004.

27. [Name redacted]. Information paper: status of charges pending against LTC [Lieutenant Colonel] ———. Dec. 4, 2003, 8093-94.

28. Wright T. LTC [Lieutenant Colonel] ———. Sep. 15, 2003, 8089-90.

29. [Unsigned Military Memo]. Information paper: status of charges pending against LTC [Lieutenant Colonel] ———. Dec. 4, 2003, 8089-90.

30. Sontag D. How colonel risked his career by menacing detainee and lost. New York Times May 27, 2004.

31. Sontag D. How colonel risked his career by menacing detainee and lost. New York Times May 27, 2004.

32. US Army: 43rd Military Police Detachment, 10th Military Police Battalion. Criminal Investigation Division Report-Final-152-03-CID469-60212. Feb. 6, 2004, DODDOACID 000111.

33. US Army, 10th Military Police Detachment, 3rd Military Police Group. CID Report of Investigation-Final (C)0031-03-CID519-62147j/5C1N /5X/15Y2D/5Y2G. Jun. 8, 2003, Taguba Annex 34.

34. Wright T. 320th MP soldiers and allegations of maltreatment of EPWs [Enemy Prisoners of War]. Sep. 15, 2003, 8090-92.

35. Marchand M. Information paper: charges pending for abuse of Iraqi detainees. Dec. 4, 2003, 8087-88.

36. Sabatino R. Deposition. Feb. 10, 2004, Taguba Annex 47:22–24.

37. Karpinski J. Sworn interview. Feb. 10, 2004, in Greenberg and Dratel, 546.

38. Sabatino R. Deposition. Feb. 10, 2004, Taguba Annex 47:24.

39. Maddocks G. Sworn interview. Feb. 14, 2004, Taguba Annex 48.

40. Maddocks G. Sworn interview. Feb. 14, 2004, Taguba Annex 48.

41. Sheridan M. Sworn statement. Feb. 14, 2004, Taguba Annex 60:9.

42. Struck D, Schneider H, Vick K, Baker P. Borderless network of terror. Washington Post Sep. 23, 2001, A1.

43. Agence France-Presse. Western intel knew Bin Laden's plan since 1995. Dec. 8, 2001.

44. Dostoevsky FM. *The Brothers Karamazov.* Garnett C (tr), Barnes & Noble Classics, NY, [first published 1879], 227.

45. Krauthammer C. The truth about torture. The Weekly Standard 2005;11:12.

46. Levinson (throughout: contains essays from various points of view).

47. Pfaff CA. Toward an ethics of detention and interrogation: consent and limits. Philosophy and Public Policy Quarterly 2005;3:18–21.

48. Allhoff F. Terrorism and torture. International Journal of Applied Philosophy 2003;17:121–34.

49. Dershowitz A. Tortured reasoning. In Levinson 257–80.

50. McCoy AW. Cruel science: CIA torture and US foreign policy. New England Journal of Public Policy 2005;19:209–62.

51. Final Report of the Senate Select Committee to Study Governmental Operations with Respect to Intelligence Activities ["Church Committee"]. 94th Cong. 2d Sess., 1976.

52. *Central Intelligence Agency et al. v. Sims et al.* 471 U.S. Supreme Court 159 (1985).

53. CIA. KUBARK Counterintelligence Interrogation Manual. Jul. 1963. [Pagination not possible, secondary to redactions.]

54. US Army. FM 34-52 Intelligence Interrogation. Washington, DC, May–Aug. 1987.

55. Segal J. Correlates of collaboration and resistance behavior among US Army POWs in Korea. Journal of Social Issues 1957;133:31–40.

56. Working Group Report on Detainee Interrogations in the Global War on Terrorism. Apr. 4, 2003, in Greenfield and Dratel 331–32, 335–37, 344–46.

57. CBS News. Memo cites captive abuse cover-up. Dec. 8, 2004.

58. Zernike K. Soldiers testify on orders to soften prisoners in Iraq. New York Times Jan. 13, 2005.

59. Mackey C, Miller G. *The Interrogators.* New York: Little, Brown, 2004, 32.

60. FBI. Transcription. Dec. 10, 2004, Detainees-3930-31.

61. FBI. Interview memo. Apr. 16, 2003, Detainees-4001-03.

62. FBI. Interview memo. Mar. 7, 2003, Detainees-3970-71.

63. FBI. Interview memo. Mar. 17, 2003, Detainees-3972-77.

64. FBI. Interview memo. Dec. 3, 2004, Detainees-3998.

65. [Sender's name redacted]. Investigation of abuse. May 20, 2004, DOD 045195-6.

66. FBI. Interview memo. Mar. 6, 2003, Detainees-3968-69.

67. Murray C. Foreign and Commonwealth Office e-mail. Receipt of intelligence obtained under torture. Jul. undated, 2004.

68. Jehl D. Qaeda-Iraq link U.S. cited is tied to coercion claim. New York Times Dec. 9, 2005.

69. Interview memo. Date redacted. Detainees-4015-16.

70. FBI. Interview memo. Mar. 19, 2003, Detainees-3978-81.

71. FBI. Interview memo. Mar. 28, 2003, Detainees-3982-84.

72. FBI. Interview memo. Mar. 19, 2003, Detainees-3985-86.

73. FBI. Interview memo. Apr. 8, 2003, Detainees-3988-89.

74. FBI. Interview memo. Apr. 8, 2003, Detainees-3989-91.

75. FBI. Interview memo. Apr. 8, 2003, Detainees-3992-95.

76. FBI. Interview memo. Apr. 9, 2003, Detainees-3996-97.

77. FBI. Interview memo. Apr. 18, 2003, Detainees-4004-86.

78. FBI. Interview memo. Apr. 21, 2003, Detainees-4008-10.

79. FBI. Interview memo. Apr. 23, 2003, Detainees-4013-15.

80. Qouta S, Punamaki RL, Sarraj EE. Prison experiences and coping styles among Palestinian men. Peace and Conflict: Journal of Peace Psychology 1997;3:19–36.

81. Afshari R. Tortured confessions. Human Rights Quarterly 2001;23: 290–97.

82. Human Rights Watch/Middle East. *Torture and Ill-Treatment: Israel's Interrogation of Palestinians from the Occupied Territories.* New York: Rights Watch, 1994.

83. Mackey C, Miller G. *The Interrogators.* New York: Little, Brown, 2004.

84. Hudson RA. The sociology and psychology of terrorism: who becomes a terrorist and why? Federal Research Division, Library of Congress, http://www.loc.gov/rr/frd/pdf-files/Soc_Psych_of_Terrorism.pdf. Accessed December 18, 2004.

85. [Name redacted, of the 470th Military Intelligence Group]. Sworn statement. May 18, 2004, DOD 000859-63.

86. Karpinski J. Deposition. Jul. 18, 2004, DOD 000089-329.

87. [Name redacted, of the 304th Military Intelligence Battalion]. Sworn statement. May 21, 2004, DOD 000598-605.

88. Fay in Greenberg and Dratel, 1042.

89. Aussaresses P. *The Battle of the Casbah: Terrorism and Counter-terrorism in Algeria 1955–1957.* New York: Enigma Books, 2002.

90. International Institute for Strategic Studies. London: Strategic Survey 2003, 2004.

91. Pew Research Center. A year after Iraq war: mistrust of America in Europe ever higher, Muslim anger persists. Pew Charitable Trusts. Washington, DC. Mar. 16, 2004.

92. Zakaria F. Pssst . . . nobody loves a torturer. Newsweek Nov. 14, 2005.

93. Working Group Report on Detainee Interrogations in the Global War on Terrorism. Apr. 4, 2003, in Greenfield and Dratel 335–36, 346.

94. Priest D. CIA puts harsh tactics on hold. Washington Post Jun. 27, 2004, A1.

95. Working Group Report on Detainee Interrogations in the Global War on Terrorism. Apr. 4, 2003, in Greenfield and Dratel, 346.

96. MacNair RM. Perpetration-induced traumatic stress in combat veterans. Peace and Conflict: Journal of Peace Psychology 2002; 8:63–67.

97. Lifton 1973, 41–71.

98. Simerman J. Soldier: leadership did little to reduce Iraqi inmate abuse. Knight Ridder Newspapers May 10, 2004.

99. Sontag S. *Regarding the Pain of Others*. New York: Farrar, Straus & Giroux, 2003, 22, 45, 90.

100. McNutt K. Sexualized Violence Against Iraqi Women by US Occupying Forces. A Briefing Paper of International Educational Development, 2005. http://psychoanalystsopposewar.org/resources_files/SVIW-1.doc.

101. Pappas T. Sworn statement. Feb. 12, 2004, Taguba Annex 46:29.

102. [Name redacted]. Personal statement to Navy Criminal Investigation Service, Camp Al Taqaddum, Iraq. Aug. 17, 2004, DODDON [Department of Defense, Department of the Navy] 000343-48.

103. Rush Limbaugh Show. It's not about us; this is war. May 4, 2004. Archived at Media Matters for America.

104. Lelyveld J. Interrogating ourselves. New York Times Magazine Jun. 12, 2005, cover, 36–43, 60, 66–69.

105. Molinski D. Colombian artist depicts Abu Ghraib abuse. Associated Press Apr. 12, 2005.

106. Wallach A. New "truisms" in words and light. New York Times Sep. 28, 2005.

107. Harvey B. In Turkish movie, Americans kill innocents. Associated Press Feb. 3, 2006.

108. Cody E. Iraqis put contempt for troops on display. Washington Post Jun. 12, 2004, A1.

CHAPTER 2: MEDICINE AND TORTURE

1. British Medical Association, 59–60.

2. Rasmussen OV. Medical aspects of torture. Danish Medical Bulletin. 1990;37 (suppl 1):1–88.

3. McCoy AW. Cruel science. New England Journal of Public Policy 1005;19:209–262.

4. Ruthven, 25–31.

5. Scott GR. *The History of Torture Through the Ages*. London: Luxor Press, 1959.

6. Langbein JH. "The Legal History of Torture," in Levinson, 93–105.

7. Maio G. History of medical involvement in torture—then and now. Lancet 2001;357:1609–1611.

8. Beccaria C. *Of Crimes and Punishments.* 1764, Chapter 16.

9. Cited at 122 in Holmes S. Is defiance of law a proof of success? In Greenberg 118–135.

10. Blackstone W. *Commentaries on the Laws of England.* Oxford: Clarendon Press, 1765, Book IV, 321.

11. Weiner DB. The real Dr. Guillotin. JAMA 1972;220:85, 88–89.

12. Amnesty International. El Salvador: Killings, Torture and Disappearances AMR 2/92, Jul. 90, 1990.

13. Reis C. Ahmed AT, Amowitz LL, et al. Physician participation in human rights abuses in southern Iraq. JAMA 2004;291:1480–86.

14. Reynolds TS, Bernstein T. Edison and the chair. IEEE Technology and Society Magazine 1989; (March):19–28.

15. Lifton 1986, 22–103.

16. Michalos C. Medical ethics and the executing process in the United States of America. Medicine and Law 1997;16:125–68.

17. Jadresic A. Doctors and torture. Journal of Medical Ethics 1980;6: 124–27.

18. Iacopino V, Heisler M, Pishevar S, et al. Physician complicity in misrepresentation and omission of evidence of torture in post-detention medical examinations in Turkey. JAMA 1996;276:396–402.

19. Chilean Medical Association. The participation of physicians in torture, in Stover E. *The Open Secret: Torture and the Medical Profession in Chile.* Washington, DC: American Association for the Advancement of Science, 1987.

20. Fisk R. Saddam's vilest prison has been swept clean, but questions remain. The Independent Sep. 17, 2003.

21. British Medical Association, 35–40.

22. Lifton 1986, 418–65.

23. Proctor RN. *Racial Hygiene: Medicine Under the Nazis.* Cambridge, Mass.: Harvard University Press, 1988.

24. Bloch S, Reddaway P. Psychiatrists and dissenters in the Soviet Union, in Stover and Nightingale, 132–63.

25. Dekleva DB, Post JM. Genocide in Bosnia: the case of Dr. Radovan

Karadzic. Journal of the American Academy of Psychiatry and Law 1997;25:485–96.

26. British Medical Association, 8.

27. Bloche MG. *Uruguay's Military Physicians: Cogs in a System of State Terror.* Washington, DC: American Association for the Advancement of Science, 1987:15.

28. Jadresic A. Doctors and torture. Journal of Medical Ethics 1980;6: 124–27.

29. Lloyd GER. *Magic, Reason, and Experience: Studies in the Origin and Development of Greek Science.* Cambridge, England: Cambridge University Press, 1979:356–60.

30. Celsus. *De Medicine.* Proemium to Book 1, 23.

31. Harris S. *Factories of Death: Japanese Biological Warfare, 1932–45, and the American Cover-up.* New York: Routledge, 2002.

32. Glendon MA. *A World Made New: Eleanor Roosevelt and the Universal Declaration of Human Rights.* New York: Random House, 2002, 235–41.

33. Annas GJ, Grodin MA (eds). *The Nazi Doctors and the Nuremberg Code: Human Rights in Human Experimentation.* New York: Oxford University Press, 1995.

34. Williams P, Wallace D. *Unit 731.* London: Grafton, 1990, 314.

35. Stover and Nightingale, 30–44, 253–79.

36. The Manual on Effective Investigation and Documentation of Torture and Other Cruel, Inhuman or Degrading Treatment or Punishment (The Istanbul Protocol), 1999.

37. American College of Physicians. The role of the physician and the medical profession in the prevention of international torture and in the treatment of its survivors. Annals of Internal Medicine 1995;122: 607–613.

38. British Medical Association 168–182.

39. Lifton RJ. Doctors and torture. New England Journal of Medicine 2004;351:415–16.

40. Sagan LA, Jonsen A. Medical ethics and torture. New England Journal of Medicine 1976;294:1427–30.

41. World Medical Association, Declaration of Tokyo [Guidelines for Med-

ical Doctors Concerning Torture and Other Cruel, Inhuman or Degrading Treatment or Punishment in Relation to Detention and Imprisonment]. Adopted by the 29th World Medical Assembly, Tokyo, Japan. Oct. 1975.

42. Amnesty International. Nurses and human rights AI Index: ACT 75/002/1997, 1997.

43. World Psychiatric Association, Declaration of Madrid. 1996.

44. Allodi FA. Assessment and treatment of torture victims: a critical review. Journal of Nervous and Mental Disease 1991;179:4–11.

45. Goldfeld AE, Mollica RF, Pesavento BH, Faraone SV. The physical and psychological sequelae of torture. Symptomatology and diagnosis. JAMA 1988;259:2725–29.

46. Shresta NM, Sharma B, Van Ommeren M, et al. Impact of torture on refugees displaced within the developing world. JAMA 1998;280: 443–48.

47. Mollica RF. Surviving torture. New England Journal of Medicine 2004;351:5–7.

48. American College of Physicians. The role of the physician and the medical profession in the prevention of international torture and in the treatment of its survivors. Annals of Internal Medicine 1995;122:607–613.

49. Joint Resolution of the American Psychiatric Association and the American Psychological Association Against Torture. Dec. 1985.

50. British Medical Association, 29, 34, 60.

51. Amnesty International. Human rights violations and the health professions. Oct. 11 1996, AI Index: AMR 19/025/1996.

52. Bloche MG. Uruguay's military physicians: cogs in a system of state terror. JAMA 1986;255:2788–93.

53. World Medical Association General Assembly. Statement on the Licensing of Physicians Fleeing Prosecution for Serious Criminal Offences. Nov. 1997.

54. Physicians for Human Rights. Sowing fear: the uses of torture and psychological abuse in Chile. 1988.

55. Physicians for Human Rights. Torture in Turkey and its unwilling accomplices. 1996.

56. Cilasun U. Torture and the participation of doctors. Journal of Medical Ethics 1991;17:21–22.

57. Amnesty International. Medical letter writing action: prosecution of doctors: Dr H Zeki Uzun. Turkey index: Jul. 7, 2002.

58. Reddaway PB. The attack on Anatoly Koryagin. New York Review of Books 1983;30(3).

59. CNN. Anatoly Koryagin. Archival news footage. Jan. 20, 1977.

60. Anonymous. Frances Ames: human rights champion. South African Medical Journal 2003;93:14–15.

61. McLean GR, Jenkins T. The Steve Biko affair: a case study in medical ethics. Developing World Bioethics 2003;3:77–95.

62. Claude RP. Torture on trial: the case of Joelito Filartiga and the Clinic of Hope, in Stover and Nightingale, 79–100.

63. Hall P. Doctors and the war on terrorism. British Medical Journal 2004;329:66.

PART II: "TANTAMOUNT TO TORTURE"

CHAPTER 3: INTERROGATION

1. McChesney J. The death of an Iraqi prisoner. National Public Radio. Oct. 27, 2005.

2. Fay in Greenberg and Dratel, 1056–1057, 1077–1078.

3. Cloud DS. Seal officer's trial gives glimpse of CIA's role in abuse. New York Times May 26, 2005.

4. Fast B. Statement. Jul. 20, 2004, DOD 00663–00670.

5. Jehl D., Golden T. CIA is likely to avoid charges in most prisoner deaths. New York Times Oct. 23, 2005.

6. Mayer J. A deadly interrogation. The New Yorker Nov. 14, 2005.

7. Hettena S. Iraqi died while hung from wrists. Associated Press Feb. 17, 2005.

8. Thomsen AB, Eriksen J, Smidt-Nielsen K. [Neurogenic pain following Palestinian hanging.] Ugeskr Laeger 1997:159:4129–30.

9. [Name redacted, of 372nd Military Police Company]. Sworn statement. May 7, 2004, DOD 000560–62.

10. Fisk R. Saddam's vilest prison has been swept clean, but questions remain. The Independent Sep. 17, 2003.

11. [Name redacted, of 372nd Military Police Company]. Sworn statement. May 4, 2004, DOD 000529–30.

12. [Name redacted, of 470th Military Intelligence Group]. Sworn statement. May 18, 2004, DOD 00340–46.

13. Harmon S. First sworn statement. Jan. 14, 2004, Taguba Annex 25/26.

14. Pappas TM. Sworn statement. May 14, 2004, DOD 000623–29.

15. Surgeon General, 20:5.

16. Church, 20–21.

17. [Name redacted, of 535th Military Intelligence Battalion]. Sworn statement. Jun. 5, 2004, DOD 000614.

18. [Name redacted, of 70th Military Intelligence Group]. Sworn statement. May 18, 2004, DOD 000340–46.

19. Armed Forces Institute of Pathology. Mon Adel Al-Jamadi: death certificate and autopsy ME 03-504. Nov. 9, 2003, MEDCOM 85–92, 177.

20. Harding K. How Abu Ghraib torture victim faces final indignity: an unmarked grave. The Guardian Jun. 1, 2004.

21. [Name redacted]. Taskers. E-mail to ALCON [all concerned]. Aug. 14, 2003, 6622–23.

22. White W. Soldiers' "wish lists" of detainee tactics cited. Washington Post Apr. 19, 2005, A16.

23. [Name redacted]. Taskers. Legal review. E-mail. Aug. 14, 2003, 6622.

24. [Name redacted]. RE: FW: Taskers. E-mail. Aug. 14, 2003, 6621.

25. [Name redacted]. E-mail RE: FW: Taskers. E-mail. Aug. 14, 2003, 6621–22.

26. [Name redacted]. Alternative Techniques (Wish List). E-mail. 4th Infantry Division, ICE. Undated. 6627–28.

27. Odierno R. Treatment of Detainees in the Custody of US Forces. Sep. 21, 2003, 002076–77 and 001807.

28. [Name redacted]. Detainee Abuse Incident-15-6 Investigation. Oct. 6, 2003, 6627–44.

29. Karpinski J. Deposition. Jul. 18, 2004, DOD 000129 (complete document is DOD 00089–325).

30. Karpinski J. Deposition. Jul. 18, 2004, DOD 000131–32.

31. Miller G. Assessment of DOD Counterterrorism Interrogation and Detention Operations in Iraq. Sep. 9, 2003, in Taguba 20 in Greenberg and Dratel, 451–59.

32. Miller G. Sworn statement. Jun. 19, 2004, DOD 000636–37.

33. Sanchez R. Combined Joint Task Forces Interrogation and Counter Resistance Policy. Oct. 12, 2003, in Greenberg and Dratel, 460–65.

34. Pappas T. Sworn statement (first interview). Feb. 9, 2004, Taguba 46.

35. [Author's name redacted.] "Training" extract [from Taguba report]. May 11, 2004, 001015–018.

36. AFOP-TRO Information Paper. Aug. 24, 2004, 001081–1085.

37. Army Inspector General in Greenberg and Dratel, 661–63, 720–29.

38. US Army. Enemy Prisoners of War, Retained Personnel, Civilian Internees and Other Detainees. Regulation 190-8, 1997, 1-5(4)e.

39. Karpinski J. Deposition. Jul. 18, 2004, DOD 148–49, 186–89, 219–23, 251–53, 277.

40. [Name redacted, of the 519th Military Intelligence Battalion]. Sworn statement. May 19, 2004, DOD 00867–71.

41. [Name redacted, of the 470th Military Intelligence Group]. Sworn statement. May 18, 2004, DOD 000859–63.

42. Karpinski J. Deposition. Jul. 18, 2004, DOD 000151.

43. [Name redacted, of the 304th Military Intelligence Battalion]. Sworn statement. May 21, 2004, DOD 000598–605.

44. Fay in Greenberg and Dratel, 1042.

45. ICRC in Greenberg and Dratel, 388.

46. [Name redacted, of Human Resources Command]. Sworn statement. May 24, 2004, DOD 000591–97.

47. Pentagon News Transcript. Special Defense Department Briefing on Results of Investigation of Military Activities at Abu Ghraib Prison Facility. Aug. 25, 2004.

48. [Name redacted, of the 519th Military Intelligence Battalion]. Sworn statement. May 19, 2004, DOD 000867–71.

49. Karpinski J. Deposition. Jul. 18, 2004, DOD 000257.

50. Karpinski J. Deposition. Jul. 18, 2004, DOD 000200.

51. [Name redacted, of 6th Military Intelligence Battalion, 98th Division]. Sworn statement. May 28, 2004, DOD 000472–473.

52. White J. US generals in Iraq were told of abuse early, inquiry finds. Washington Post Dec. 1, 2004, A1.

53. Shanker T. Abu Ghraib called incubator for terrorists. New York Times Feb. 15, 2006.

54. Army Inspector General in Greenberg and Dratel, 675.

55. Joint Interrogation and Debriefing Center. Interrogation Rules of Engagement (IROE). Jan. 23, 2004, Taguba Annex 40:26–28.

56. Petosky E. Air Force medics aid Abu Ghraib prisoners. 332 Air Expeditionary Wing. Armed Forces News Service May 11, 2005.

57. Surgeon General, 11:1–3.

58. [Name redacted, of the 519th Military Intelligence Battalion]. Sworn statement. May 19, 2004, DOD 000867–71.

59. Tudor J. Airmen provide exams before, after interrogations. Air Force News Jul. 27, 2005.

60. US Army, Criminal Investigation Command, 3rd Military Police Group. CID Report of Investigation. Final C-SSI-0149-04-CID259-80212-/5C1R/25Y2E5X1. Aug. 3, 2004, DODDOACID 001458–508.

61. Miller G (Major General). Assessment of DOD Counterterrorism Interrogation and Detention Operations in Iraq. Sep. 9, 2003, in Taguba 20 in Greenberg and Dratel, 451–59.

62. Secretary of Defense. Memorandum for the Commander, US Southern Command; Counter Resistance Techniques in the War on Terrorism. Apr. 16, 2003, in Greenberg and Dratel, 360–65.

63. Surgeon General, 1:8.

64. Surgeon General, 18:12.

65. Mayer J. The experiment. The New Yorker Jul. 11, 2005, 60–71.

66. Joint Interrogation and Debriefing Center. Organizational Chart. Jan. 23, 2004, Taguba Annex 40:18.

67. Program notes for American Academy of Psychiatry and the Law 2004, annual meeting, list Dr. Uithol as an invited speaker on forensic psychiatric issues in a combat zone.

68. Stratford B. Combating combat stress in Iraq. Anaconda Times (Baghdad) Mar. 8, 2004, 4.

69. Bloche MG, Marks JH. Doctors and interrogators at Guantánamo Bay. New England Journal of Medicine 2005;353;1:6–8.

70. AMEDD. Aeromedical Policy Letter. Mar. 5, 2002.

71. Bloche MG, Marks JH. Doctors and interrogators at Guantánamo Bay. New England Journal of Medicine 2005;353;1:6–8.

72. Mayer J. The experiment. The New Yorker Jul. 11, 2005, 60–71.

73. United States Southern Command. Policy Memorandum 8-01 US

Southern Command Confidentiality Policy for Interactions Between Health Care Providers and Enemy Persons Under US Control, Detained in Conjunction with Operation Enduring Freedom. Aug. 6, 2002.

74. Surgeon General, 18:13.

75. Slevin P, Stephens J. Detainees' medical files shared: Guantanamo interrogators' access criticized. Washington Post Jun. 10, 2004: A1.

76. Lewis N. Red Cross finds detainee abuse in Guantánamo. New York Times Nov. 20, 2004.

77. Surgeon General, 1:4.

78. [Name redacted] Debriefer/Interrogator to Chief. Witnessing of harsh treatment to Iraqi detainees held in camp Na'ma. May 8, 2004, DODDOACID 009145–46.

79. Snider S. Sworn statement. Feb. 12, 2004, Taguba 84.

80. Slevin P, Stephens J. Detainees' medical files shared: Guantanamo interrogators' access criticized. Washington Post Jun. 10, 2004: A1.

81. [Name redacted, of the 470th Military Intelligence Group]. Sworn statement. May 18, 2004, DOD 000340–46.

82. Stefanowicz (aka Stephanowicz) S. Sworn statement. Jun. 22, 2004, Taguba Annex 25/26 in Greenberg and Dratel, 475–76, and Taguba Annex 90:2, 28–31, 40–41.

83. Mayer J. The experiment. The New Yorker Jul. 11, 2005, 60–71.

84. Pappas TM. Request for Exception to CJTF Interrogation and Counter Resistance Policy. Nov. 30, 2003, in Greenberg and Dratel, 466–67.

85. Pappas T. Sworn statement. Feb. 11, 2004, Taguba 46.

86. Karpinski J. Deposition. Jul. 18, 2004, DOD 000089–325.

87. Miller G. Sworn statement. Jun. [redacted] 2004, DOD 000640–41.

88. [Name redacted, of 500th Military Intelligence Group]. Memorandum for the Record. Jun. 9, 2004, DOD 000391–94.

89. [Name redacted, of 304th Military Intelligence Battalion]. Sworn statement. May 21, 2004, DOD 000598–605.

90. [Name redacted, of Human Resources Command]. Sworn statement. May 24, 2004, DOD 591–95.

91. [Name redacted, of 470th Military Intelligence Group]. May 18, 2004, DOD 000340–46.

92. Pappas T. Sworn statement. Feb. 11, 2004, Taguba Annex 46.

93. Elliot R. Sworn statement. Feb. 12, 2004, Taguba Annex 86.

94. Comer K. Sworn statement. Feb. 10, 2004, Taguba Annex 85.

95. [Unnamed author]. Abu Ghraib Bullet Report. Jul. 12, 2004, 008168–76.

96. [Unnamed author]. Joint Interrogation & Debriefing Center, Abu Ghurayb, Iraq. Briefing Slides. Taguba Annex 40.

97. Secretary of Defense. Memorandum for the Commander, US Southern Command; Counter Resistance Techniques in the War on Terrorism. Apr. 16, 2003, in Greenberg and Dratel, 360–65.

98. Miller G. Assessment of DOD Counterterrorism Interrogation and Detention Operations in Iraq. Sep. 9, 2003, in Greenberg and Dratel, 453, 455.

99. Sanchez R. Combined Joint Task Forces Interrogation and Counter Resistance Policy. Oct. 12, 2003, in Greenberg and Dratel, 460–61.

100. Army Bravo Company, 311 Military Intelligence Battalion, Mosul Iraq. Instructions for guard force assigned to 2nd Brigade holding area. Nov. 14, 2003, 001334–346.

101. Stefanowicz (aka Stephanowicz) S. Sworn statement. Jun. 22, 2004, Taguba Annex 25/26, in Greenberg and Dratel, 475–76.

102. Snider S. Sworn statement. Feb. 12, 2004, Taguba Annex 84.

103. Army Inspector General in Greenberg and Dratel, 666–68.

104. Taguba Executive Summary in Greenberg and Dratel, 410.

105. Wojdakowski W. Corrective actions required after riots and shootings at Abu Ghraib prison on 24 November 2003. [date redacted], Taguba Annex 8.

106. Higham S, Stephens J. Punishment and amusement. Washington Post May 22, 2004, A1.

107. Secretary of Defense. Memorandum for the Commander, US Southern Command; Counter Resistance Techniques in the War on Terrorism. Apr. 16, 2003, in Greenberg and Dratel, 360–65.

108. Sanchez R. Combined Joint Task Forces Interrogation and Counter Resistance Policy. Oct. 12, 2003, in Greenberg and Dratel, 460–65.

109. Pappas T. Sworn statement. Feb. 14, 2004, Taguba Annex 46:4–5.

110. Bloche MG, Marks JH. Doctors and interrogators at Guantanamo Bay. New England Journal of Medicine 2005; 353;1:6–8.

111. Stefanowicz (aka Stephanowicz) S. Sworn statement. Taguba Annex 25/26 in Greenberg and Dratel, 475–76.

112. [Name redacted, of the 519th Military Intelligence Battalion]. Sworn statement. May 19, 2004, DOD 000867–71.

113. [Name redacted, of Combined Joint Special Operation Task Force–Arabian Peninsula]. Sworn statement of command psychologist. Jul. 12, 2004. DODDOACID 000558.

114. 43rd Military Policy Detachment, 22 Military Police. CID Report of Investigation-Final C-0139-03-CID469-60206-5YEFeb. 5Y2PSep. 9G1. Oct. 13, 2004, DODDOACID 008809–9008 at 008818–27.

115. Surgeon General, 20:9.

116. Mayer J. The experiment. The New Yorker Jul. 1, 2005, 60–71.

117. Surgeon General, 18:14, 20:8.

118. Zagorin A, Duffy M. Inside the interrogation of detainee 063. Time Jun. 20, 2005, 26–33.

119. Bloche MG, Marks JH. Doctors and interrogators at Guantanamo Bay. New England Journal of Medicine 2005;353;1:6–8.

120. Bashour TT, Gualberto A, Ryan C. Atrioventricular block in accidental hypothermia—a case report. Angiology 1989;40:63–66.

121. Gould L, Gopalaswamy C, Kim BS, et al. The Osborn wave in hypothermia. Angiology 1985;36:125–29.

122. Furlow JT. Final Report Investigation into FBI Allegations of Detainee Abuse at Guantanamo Bay, Cuba Detention Facility. Jun. 9, 2005, 17.

123. Rumsfeld D. Counter Resistance Techniques. Nov. 27, 2002, in Greenberg and Dratel, 237.

124. Rumsfeld D. Counter Resistance Techniques. Jan. 15, 2002, in Greenberg and Dratel, 239.

125. Kozaryn LD. Al Qaeda leader Zubaydah to remain in US control. Armed Forces Press Service Apr. 3, 2002.

126. Priest D. CIA puts harsh tactics on hold. Washington Post Jun. 27, 2004, A1.

127. Bonner R, Van Natta D, Waldman A. Questioning terror suspects in a dark and surreal world. New York Times Mar. 9, 2003.

128. Priest D, Gellman B. US decries abuse but defends interrogations. Washington Post Dec. 26, 2002.

129. [Name and unit redacted]. AR 15-6 Investigation. Sworn statement. Oct. 1, 2003, 6630.

130. US Army, Criminal Investigation Command. CID Final Report of Investigation. Dec. 28, 2004 DODDOACID 008604–008762.

131. *Al-Laithi S et al. v. George Walker Bush et al.*, cvi no 05cv429, US District Court for District of Columbia, filed July 21, 2005.

132. FBI. Interview memo. Sep. 5, 2002, Detainees-3894-95.

133. FBI. Interview memo. Jul. 2, 2003, Detainees-4051-53.

134. Saar and Viveca, 73–74.

135. Mayer J. The experiment. The New Yorker Jul. 11, 2005, 60–71.

136. Surgeon General, 11:1–3

137. Tudor J. Airmen provide exams before, after interrogations. Air Force News Jul. 27, 2005.

138. Stephens S. Army doctors implicated in abuse. Washington Post Jan. 6, 2005, A6.

139. Winkenwerder W, Kiley KC, Arthur DC, et al. Doctors and torture. New England Journal of Medicine 2005;351:1572–73.

140. White J. Review calls abuse cases isolated. Washington Post Jul. 8, 2005, A21.

141. Bloche MG, Marks JH. When doctors go to war. New England Journal of Medicine 2004;352:3–6.

142. Department of Justice. Inmate physical and mental health record system. Federal Register Mar. 15, 2002;67(51):11712–14.

143. Bloche MG, Marks JH. Doctors and interrogators at Guantanamo Bay. New England Journal of Medicine 2005;353;1:6–8.

144. Assistant Secretary of Defense. Medical Program Principles and Procedures for the Protection and Treatment of Detainees in the Custody of the Armed Forces of the United States. Jun. 3, 2005.

145. Rhem KT. DoD issues guidance for medical personnel dealing with detainees. Armed Forces Information Service. Jun. 16, 2005.

146. Rubenstein L, Pross C, Davidoff F, et al. Coercive US interrogation policies: a challenge to medical ethics. JAMA 205;294:1544–49.

147. Surgeon General, 18:17–22.

148. Kiley KC. Memorandum for Record (Attached to Surgeon General, Report) May 24, 2005.

149. Church, 19–20.

150. Peterson HD. Torture in a democratic country, 1989. Danish Medical Bulletin 1990;37:556–59.

151. Lewis N. Red Cross finds detainee abuse in Guantánamo. New York Times Nov. 20, 2004.
152. British Medical Association. Handbook of Medical Ethics. 1984, 44.

CHAPTER 4: HOMICIDE

1. Golden T. The Bagram file. New York Times May 20, 2005. (Facts came from government documents held by New York Times that are not available to public.)
2. Golden T. Army faulted in investigating detainee abuse. New York Times May 22, 2005. (Facts come from government files held by New York Times that are not available to public.)
3. Final Report of Post-mortem Examination Armed Forces Regional Medical Examiner. Dec. 6–8, 2002, MEDCOM 19–27.
4. Golden T. Abuse inquiry opens questions of army tactics. New York Times Aug. 8, 2005.
5. Armed Forces Institute of Pathology. Dilawar: autopsy No. A02-95. Dec. 13, 2002, MEDCOM 29–36.
6. Gall C, Rohde D. New charges raise questions on abuse in Afghan prisons. New York Times Sep. 17, 2004.
7. Gall C, Rohde D. New charges raise questions on abuse in Afghan prisons. New York Times Sep. 17, 2004.
8. Gall C. U.S. Military investigating death of Afghan in custody. New York Times Mar. 4, 2003.
9. Armed Forces Institute of Pathology. Dilawar: death certificate (downloaded from DoD website, no longer posted).
10. Armed Forces Institute of Pathology. Dilawar: death certificate Dec. 13, 2002, MEDCOM 169.
11. Armed Forces Institute of Pathology. Fahin Al Gunna: death certificate. Jun. 2, 2004, MEDCOM 175.
12. Golden T. Years after 2 Afghans died, abuse case falters. New York Times, Feb. 13, 2006.
13. Church, 20–21.
14. An earlier version of this chapter was published as Miles SH. Medical investigations of homicides of prisoners of war in Iraq and Afghanistan. MedScape 2005;7(3).

15. [Name redacted, staff of Criminal Investigation Task Force]. After action report: preliminary investigation into the death of a detainee at Geresceh forward operating base, Helmand Province, Afghanistan. Approx Dec. 2003, DOD 045198.

16. ICRC in Greenberg and Dratel, 398–99.

17. Taguba Annex 10.

18. Armed Forces Medical Examiner System, Army Regulation 40–57. Jan. 2, 1991.

19. Clark MA, Ruehle CJ, Wright DG, et al. The armed forces' medical examiner system: a change for the better. Aviation Space & Environmental Medicine 1989:60(7 Pt 2):A1,3.

20. Weedn V. The potential federal role in the death investigation system. Institute of Medicine Workshop 2003.

21. World Medical Association. Resolution on the Responsibility of Physicians in the Denunciation of Acts of Torture or Cruel or Inhuman or Degrading Treatment of Which They Are Aware. Helsinki 2003.

22. Department of Defense. Background Briefing by Senior Military Official and Senior Pentagon Medical Official. http://www.defenselink.mil/transcripts/2004/tr20040521-0791.html, May 21, 2004.

23. Department of Defense. Death certificates of Dilawar, Abdul Wahid, and Habibullah are available at http://www.defenselink.mil/news/May2004/d20040521cert.pdf.

24. Department of Defense. Death Certificates of Mohammed Tariq Zaid, Hussein Awad Al-Jawadi, Ekab Ahmed Hassan, Mohammed Abdullah Saad, Mohammed Basim Hassan, Hazaad Hamza Twfeek Najm Byaty Al Zubydy, Nasef Ibrahim, Mohammed Abdul Abbas, Al-Hussen Bakir Yassen Rashad, Mohammed Najem Abed, Ehad Kazem Taled, Dham Spah, Mindy Wathik, Fahin Ali Gumaa, Abdul Jaleel, Mon Adel Al-Jamadi, Dilar Ababa, Abid Mowhoush, Naem Sadoon Hatab, and Mohammed Fashad are available at http://www.defenselink.mil/news/May2004/d20040521cert1.pdf.

25. Armed Forces Institute of Pathology. Abid Hamed Mowosh: death certificate. Redacted signature version at MEDCOM 178.

26. Armed Forces Institute of Pathology. Dham Spah: death certificate. Redacted signature version at MEDCOM 189.

27. Armed Forces Institute of Pathology. Taled Ehad Kazam: death certificate. Redacted signature version at MEDCOM 190.

28. Armed Forces Institute of Pathology. Mindy Wathik: death certificate. Redacted signature version at MEDCOM 188.

29. Armed Forces Institute of Pathology. Zaid Mohamed Tariq: death certificate. Oct. 23, 2003, MEDCOM 181.

30. [Sender's name redacted, of Navy Criminal Investigation Service]. E-mail correspondence EPW [enemy prisoner of war] Issues. May 26–Jun. 4, 2004, 3769–88.

31. Army CID, 43rd Military Police. CID Report of Investigation-Final C-0149-03-CID469-60209-5H1A. Nov. 23, 2003, 01054–181.

32. US v [Name redacted]-4ID. [Correction of CID Investigation.] 8063–84.

33. Informal investigation of shooting death of Obeed Hethere Radad under auspices of AR 15-6. Sep. 2003, DOD 044873–983.

34. Levy A, Scott-Clark C. One huge US jail. The Guardian Mar. 19, 2005.

35. Harding L. "I will always hate you people": family's fury at mystery death. The Guardian May 24, 2004.

36. Moffeit M. Skipped autopsies in Iraq revealed. Denver Post May 21, 2004.

37. Army Criminal Investigation Command, 3rd Military Police Group. CID Report of Investigation-Final/SSI-0237-04-CID259-80273-5H9B. Oct. 18, 2004, DODDOACID 004153–189.

38. Surgeon General, 20-5.

39. Pyes C, Mazzetti M. US probing alleged abuse of Afghans. Los Angeles Times Sep. 21, 2004.

40. Human Rights Watch. An Open Letter to US Secretary of Defense Donald Rumsfeld. Dec. 13, 2004.

41. Amnesty International. Iraq: Memorandum on Concerns Relating to Law and Order MDE 14/157/2003. Jul. 23, 2003, 23.

42. Surgeon General, 20-7.

43. [Name redacted, of DMAIN {Division main command post} Staff Judge Advocate's Office]. Transmittal Record: Legal Actions. Sep. 21, 2003, DOD 044867.

44. Mayer J. Annals of justice: outsourcing torture. The New Yorker Feb. 14, 2005, 106–123.

45. Kiley K. Readers' response to "Medical investigations of homicides of prisoners of war in Iraq and Afghanistan." Medscape 2005;7(3).

46. Turner SA, Barnard JJ, Spotswood SD, et al. "Homicide by heart attack" revisited. Journal of Forensic Sciences 2004;49:598–600.

47. Stalnikowicz R, Tsafrir A. Acute psychosocial stress and cardiovascular events. American Journal of Emergency Medicine 2002;20:488–91.

48. Lecomte D, Fornes P, Nicolas G. Stressful events as a trigger of sudden death: a study of 43 medico-legal autopsy cases. Forensic Science International 1996;79:1–10.

49. Appels A, Otten F. Exhaustion as precursor of cardiac death. British Journal Clinical Psychology 1992;31:351–56.

50. Wittstein IS, Thiemann DR, Lima JAC, et al. Neurohumoral features of myocardial stunning due to sudden emotional stress. New England Journal of Medicine 2005;352:539–48.

51. [Sender and recipient names redacted]. Army e-mail: Weekend Incidents in Iraq. Jun. 25, 2004, 3830.

52. Human Rights Watch. An Open Letter to US Secretary of Defense Donald Rumsfeld. Dec. 13, 2004.

53. Christian Peacemaker Team. Report on Iraqi Detainees. Sep. 24, 2004.

54. Army Criminal Investigation Command, 75th Military Police Detachment. CID Report of Investigation-Final/SSI-0059-04-CID789-83991-5H9A. Oct. 15, 2004, DODDOACID 006022–39.

55. ICRC in Greenberg and Dratel, 397.

56. Armed Forces Institute of Pathology. Zaid Mohamed Tariq: death certificate and autopsy ME-03-367. Oct. 23, 2003, MEDCOM 65–70, 181.

57. US Army, 38th Military Police Detachment, 22nd Military Police Battalion. CID Report of Investigation-Initial/Final C/SSI-0168-04-CID899-81718-5H8. May 31, 2004, 02206–215.

58. US Army re-examines deaths of Iraqi prisoners. USA Today Jun. 28 2004.

59. Armed Forces Institute of Pathology. Nasef Ibrahim: death certificate. Death Jan. 11, 2004 [death certificate finalized May 13, 2004], MEDCOM 191.

60. Armed Forces Institute of Pathology. Nasef Ibrahim: autopsy ME04-12. Jan. 11, 2004.

61. USA Today. Documents give different explanation for inmate's death. Jun. 28, 2004.

62. Army Criminal Investigation Command, 78th Military Police Detachment, 3rd Military Police Group. CID Report of Investigation-Final/Supplemental/SSI Report-0007-04-CID259-80133-5H9A. Aug. 23, 2004, 01443-79.

63. US Army, 101st Airborne, Mosul. AR 15-6 Investigation into the death of Abu Malik Kenami. Dec. 28, 2003, 001281–333.

64. US Army, 31st Military Police Detachment, 3rd Military Police Group. CID Report of Investigation-Final-0140-03-CID389-61697-5H9B. Jan. 1, 2004, 01206–219, 1351–66.

65. Armed Forces Institute of Pathology. Abdureda Lafta Abdul Kareem: death certificate and autopsy ME04-434. Oct. 13, 2004, MEDCOM 1046–1062.

66. Armed Forces Institute of Pathology. [Name redacted]: death certificate and autopsy ME04-386. Jun. 1, 2004, MEDCOM 606, 662–72.

67. Rumsfeld D. Memorandum for Secretaries of the Military Departments. Procedures for the Investigations of Deaths of Detainees in the Custody of Armed Forces of the United States. Jun. 9, 2004.

68. Media Corp News. US Army doctors implicated in Iraqi prisoner abuse scandal. Aug. 21, 2004.

69. Kiley K. Military medicine and human rights. Lancet 2004;364:1852.

70. Kiley K. Readers' response to "Medical investigations of homicides of prisoners of war in Iraq and Afghanistan." MedScape 2005;7(3).

71. Army Regulations 190-8:6–14(5–6).

72. Gilmore GJ. Medical personnel didn't commit widespread detainee abuse, says DoD. Armed Forces Information Service Feb. 11, 2005.

73. Mallak CT. [letter.] New England Journal of Medicine 2004;351:1572.

74. Myers SL. Military completed death certificates for 20 prisoners only after months passed. New York Times May 31, 2004.

75. Fisk R. British soldiers kicked Iraqi prisoner to death. The Independent Jan. 4, 2003.

76. ICRC in Greenberg and Dratel, 390.

77. US detainee death toll hits 108. BBC News Apr. 28, 2005.

78. Church, 20–21.

79. Thomsen JL. The role of the pathologist in human rights abuses. Journal of Clinical Pathology 2000;53:569–72.

80. World Medical Association. Resolution on the Responsibility of Physicians in the Denunciation of Acts of Torture or Cruel or Inhuman or Degrading Treatment of Which They Are Aware. Helsinki 2003.

81. AFRD-PM. Procedures following the death of a detainee in CFLCC [Coalition Forces Land Component Command] custody. Jan. 2, 2002, 009662.

82. Kiley K. Readers' response to "Medical investigations of homicides of prisoners of war in Iraq and Afghanistan." MedScape 2005;7(3).

83. 18 United States Code, Part I, Chapter 1 §3: Accessory After the Fact.

84. White J. Documents tell of brutal improvisation by GIs. Washington Post Aug. 3, 2005.

85. Article 32 investigation. *United States v CW2 Williams, SFC Sommer, and SPC Loper.* Dec. 2, 2004, 95–97, 238, 240.

86. Article 32 investigation, *United States v CW2 Williams, SFC Sommer, and SPC Loper.* Dec. 2, 2004, 110–111.

87. Schmitt E. Army interrogator convicted in death of Iraqi general. New York Times Jan. 22, 2006.

88. Article 32 investigation, *United States v CW2 Williams, SFC Sommer, and SPC Loper.* Dec. 2, 2004, 100–103.

89. Article 32 investigation, *United States v CW2 Williams, SFC Sommer, and SPC Loper.* Dec. 2, 2004, 96–98.

90. Article 32 investigation, *United States v CW2 Williams, SFC Sommer, and SPC Loper.* Dec. 2, 2004, 233–35, 239, 240–41.

91. Article 32 investigation, *United States v CW2 Williams, SFC Sommer, and SPC Loper.* Dec. 2, 2004, 99–100, 109, 123–25, 138–43, 163, 167–68, 186, 208–210.

92. Moffeit M. Brutal interrogation in Iraq. Denver Post May 19, 2004.

93. Armed Forces Institute of Pathology. Abed Mowhoush: death certificate and autopsy ME03-571. Dec. 2, 2003, MEDCOM 93–100, 178.

94. ICRC in Greenberg and Dratel, 389.

95. Fisher I. Searing uncertainty for Iraqi's missing loved one. New York Times Jun. 1, 2004.

96. Armed Forces Institute of Pathology Operations. Number 5154.30. Mar. 18, 2003.

97. Hettena S. Army pathologist concedes errors in prisoner-abuse case. Associated Press Oct. 14, 2004.

98. Hettena S. Errors in Iraq abuse case raise concerns. News.Orb6.com Oct. 31, 2004.

99. Article 32 investigation, *United States v CW2 Williams, SFC Sommer, and SPC Loper.* Dec. 2, 2004, 153–55.

100. Human Rights Watch. An Open Letter to US Secretary of Defense Donald Rumsfeld. Dec. 13, 2004.

101. Human Rights Watch. Afghanistan: killing and torture by US predate Abu Ghraib. May 20, 2005.

102. Jehl D, Golden T. CIA is likely to avoid charges in most prisoner deaths. New York Times Oct. 23, 2005.

103. Armed Forces Medical Examiner. Habibullah: Final Report of Post Mortem Examination CIV 011(49)6371-86-7492 A02-93. Dec. 6–8, 2002, MEDCOM 19–27.

104. Melone R. Sworn statement. Army Criminal Investigation Command, File # 0134002 CID 369-23533. Aug. 5, 2004, unpaginated].

105. Armed Forces Regional Medical Examiner. Final Report of Post Mortem Examination, CIV. 011(49)6371-86-7492. Dec. 6–8, 2002, MEDCOM 19–27.

106. Church, 20–21.

107. United States Army. Criminal Investigation Command. Criminal investigators outline 27 confirmed or suspected detainee homicides for Operation Iraqi Freedom, Operation Enduring Freedom. Mar. 25, 2005.

108. Golden T. The Bagram file. New York Times May 20, 2005.

109. Pyes C, Mazzetti M. US probing alleged abuse of Afghans. Los Angeles Times Sep. 21, 2004.

110. Department of Justice [press release]. CIA contractor indicted for assaulting detainee held at U.S. base in Afghanistan. Jun. 17, 2004.

111. Witt A. US probes death of prisoner in Afghanistan. Washington Post Jun. 24, 2003.

112. Armed Forces Institute of Pathology. Abdul Wahid: death certificate and autopsy A03-144. Nov. 13, 2003, MEDCOM 44–50, 171.

113. Human Rights Watch. An Open Letter to US Secretary of Defense Donald Rumsfeld. Dec. 13, 2004.

114. Amnesty International. Iraq: Memorandum on concerns relating to law and order [MDE 14/157/2003]. Jun. 23, 2003, 13.

115. Ehrenreich B. The torture files: Iraqi detainees allege mistreatment and abuse. LA Weekly Feb. 6–12, 2004.

116. Sherwell P, Freeman C. Iraqi prisoner was beaten, kicked and left to die by Marines. Telegraph May 23, 2004.

117. Mortenson D. Medic says Pittman hit, slapped inmates. North County (Calif.) Times Aug. 31, 2004.

118. Armed Forces Institute of Pathology. Nagen Sadoon Hatab: death certificate and autopsy A03-51. Jun. 10, 2003, MEDCOM 37–44, 174.

119. Armed Forces Institute of Pathology. Dilar Dababa: death certificate and autopsy ME03-273. May 11, 2004, MEDCOM 56–64, 179.

120. ICRC in Greenberg and Dratel, 390.

121. Fisk R. British soldiers kicked Iraqi prisoner to death. The Independent Jan. 4, 2003.

122. Amnesty International. Iraq: Amnesty International reveals a pattern of torture and ill-treatment. May 2004.

123. Amnesty International. Action appeal Iraq: Iraqi held by UK troops dies in custody. Dec. 2003.

124. Fisk R. The British said my son would be free soon. The Independent Jan. 4, 2004.

125. ICRC in Greenberg and Dratel, 390.

126. Armed Forces Institute of Pathology. Mohamed Tariq Zaid: death certificate and autopsy ME 03-367. Aug. 25, 2003, MEDCOM 65–70, 181.

127. Squitieri T, Moniz D. A third of detainees who died were assaulted. USA Today May 31, 2004.

128. US Army re-examines deaths of Iraqi prisoners. USA Today Jun. 28, 2004.

129. US v [redacted]-4ID. [Correction of CID Investigation]. 8063-84.

130. Informal investigation of shooting death of Obeed Hethere Radad under auspices of AR 15-6. DOD 044873–983.

131. Army CID, 43rd Military Police. CID Report of Investigation-Final C-0149-03-CID469-60209-5H1A. Nov. 23, 2003, 01054–1181.

132. Amnesty International. Action appeal Iraq: Iraqi held by UK troops dies in custody. Dec. 2003.

133. Fisk R. The British said my son would be free soon. The Independent Jan. 4, 2004.

134. Human Rights Watch. The road to Abu Ghraib. Jun. 2004.

135. Army Criminal Investigations Command. Army criminal investigators outline 27 confirmed or suspected detainee homicides for Operation Iraqi Freedom, Operation Enduring Freedom. Mar. 25, 2005.

136. Armed Forces Institute of Pathology. Jaleel Abdul: death certificate. May 13, 2004, MEDCOM 180.

137. White J. Three more Navy SEALs face abuse charges. Washington Post Sep. 25, 2004, A16.

138. Army Criminal Investigations Command. Army criminal investigators outline 27 confirmed or suspected detainee homicides for Operation Iraqi Freedom, Operation Enduring Freedom. Mar. 25, 2005.

139. Armed Forces Institute of Pathology. Mohamed Fashad: death certificate and autopsy ME-4-309. Apr. 5, 2004, MEDCOM 133–34, 173.

CHAPTER 5: NEGLECT

1. England L. Sworn statement. Jan. 14, 2004, in Taguba Annex 25/26, 1.
2. Surgeon General, 20-12.
3. Bloche MG, Marks JH. Triage at Abu Ghraib. New York Times Feb. 5, 2005.
4. Surgeon General, 20-12.
5. Wallin N. Sworn statement. Jan. 26, 2004, in Greenberg and Dratel, 472.
6. Ryder, 1.
7. Ryder, 37.
8. Ryder, 43.
9. Ryder, 43.
10. Ryder, 38.
11. Ryder, 38.
12. Ryder, 38.
13. Ryder, 37.
14. Army Inspector General in Greenberg and Dratel, 705, 712.
15. Army Inspector General in Greenberg and Dratel, 648.
16. Army Inspector General in Greenberg and Dratel, 660–62, 692–93, 705–774, 731–32.

17. Petosky E. Air Force medics aid Abu Ghraib prisoners. Iraq Newslink: 332 Expeditionary Wing [undated press release].

18. Fisk R. Saddam's vilest prison has been swept clean, but questions remain. The Independent Sep. 17, 2003.

19. Reis C, Ahmed AT, Amowitz LL, et al. Physician participation in human rights abuses in southern Iraq. JAMA 2004;291:1480–86.

20. Nadeau A. Proctor native in Abu Ghraib keeps hope with help of family. Proctor Journal (Minn.) Aug. 20, 2004.

21. [Name and unit redacted, cover sheet of investigation file not available]. Multiple sworn statements describing incident at Camp Whitehorse on Aug. 13, 2003. Statements collected Aug. 14–16, 2003, 6318–39, 54–56.

22. US Army, 418th Civil Affairs Battalion. Prisoner Death Investigation. Aug. 2, 2003, 6241–312.

23. Surgeon General, 20-10-11.

24. Surgeon General, 20-10-12, 18:4–6.

25. Surgeon General, 20-10-11.

26. Human Rights Watch Report. Enduring Freedom: Abuses by US Forces in Afghanistan. Mar. 2004, 39.

27. ICRC in Greenberg and Dratel, 391.

28. Army Inspector General in Greenberg and Dratel, 692–93.

29. Surgeon General, 6-1-4, 8-1-5.

30. Fay in Greenberg and Dratel, 1051, 1111, 1082.

31. CJTF7-TF-FAY. Telephone Interview—Memorandum for the Record Jun. 9, 2004, DOD 000609.

32. US Army Criminal Investigation Command, 3rd Military Police. CID Report of Investigation-Final-0189-04-CID259-80233-/5C2B/5Y2E/5X1/5M3A. Jul. 20, 2004.

33. Extensive MEDCOM clinical records from the Abu Ghraib hospital were available from the ACLU website archives as of April–May 2005.

34. Surgeon General, 20-7-8.

35. Surgeon General, 20-7.

36. Taguba Annex 103.

37. Human Rights Watch Briefing. Guantanamo: Detainee Accounts. Oct. 26, 2004, 16.

38. [Name redacted, of 470th Military Intelligence Group]. May 18, 2004, DOD 000340–46.

39. Surgeon General, 20:8.

40. World Health Organization. Tuberculosis Department 2006. http://www.who.int/tb/en/.

41. Dye C, Espinal MA, Watt C, et al. Worldwide incidence of multidrug-resistant tuberculosis. Journal of Infectious Diseases 2002;185:1197–202.

42. Conin R, Mathieu C, Debacker M, et al. First-line tuberculosis therapy and drug-resistant Mycobacterium tuberculosis in prisons. Lancet 1999;353:969–73.

43. Levy MH, Reys H, Conin R. Overwhelming consumption in prisons: human rights and tuberculosis control. Health and Human Rights 1999;4:167–91.

44. Stern V. Problems in prisons worldwide, with a particular focus on Russia. Annals of New York Academy of Science 2001;953:113–19.

45. 530th Military Police Battalion. Criminal Detainee Reception and In-Processing Standard Operating Procedure [Camp Bucca]. [Undated], Taguba Annex 16.

46. Armed Forces Institute of Pathology. Mohammed Hussain Basim: death certificate and autopsy. 03-349-B. Jul. 13, 2003, MEDCOM 51–55, 185, 674–79, 984–85.

47. Army Criminal Investigation Command, 307th Military Police Detachment. CID Report of Investigation-Final/supplemental 0014-03-CID919-73732. Jul. 21, 2004, 02060–2095.

48. Army Pamphlet 40-11. Preventive Medicine. Appendix C: Tuberculosis Surveillance and Control Guidelines.

49. Surgeon General, 20-7.

50. Miller GD. Assessment of DoD counterterrorism interrogation and detention operations in Iraq. Sep. 9, 2003, in Greenberg and Dratel, 456.

51. Army Inspector General in Greenberg and Dratel, 712.

52. U.S. Department of State. Improved conditions at Shiberghan prison. Apr. 2003 in Greenberg and Dratel, 1177–80.

53. Surgeon General, 18-5.

54. Reese D. Sworn statement. Taguba Annex 63.

55. FBI Counter Terrorism Division. Inquiry regarding activities of FBI personnel at Abu Ghurayb Prison. May 17, 2004, Detainees-1179-1190.

56. Bloche MG, Marks JH. Triage at Abu Ghraib. New York Times Feb. 5, 2005.

57. Ryder, 43.

58. Yee, 100–104.

59. ICRC in Greenberg and Dratel, 393.

60. Ryder, 43.

61. Surgeon General, 18-5-6: 20-7.

62. Army Inspector General in Greenberg and Dratel, 712.

63. Miller GD. Assessment of DoD counterworks interrogation and detention operations in Iraq. Sep. 9, 2003, in Greenberg and Dratel, 456.

64. Emergency Care and Treatment. Mosul, Dec. 24, 2003, MEDCOM 369.

65. Fay in Greenberg and Dratel, 1080.

66. Wallin N. Sworn statement Jan. 26, 2004, in Greenberg and Dratel, 472.

67. Jordan S. Interview. Taguba Annex 53, 158.

68. Jordan S. Sworn statement. Feb. 21, 2004, Taguba Annex 53:158–59.

69. Spencer L. Sworn statement. Jan. 21, 2004, Taguba Annex 25/26 in Greenberg and Dratel, 477.

70. Surgeon General, 20:14.

71. Saar and Viveca, 101–102.

72. Golden T. In U.S. report, brutal details of 2 Afghan inmates' deaths. New York Times May 20, 2005.

73. Saar and Viveca, 66, 103–104, 243.

74. Yee, 102–104.

75. Bonner R. Terror suspect's ordeal in US custody. New York Times Dec. 18, 2005.

76. White J. Guantanamo desperation seen in suicide attempts. Washington Post Nov. 1, 2005, A1.

77. Ehrenreich B. The torture files: Iraqi detainees allege mistreatment and abuse. LA Weekly Feb. 6–12, 2004.

78. Amnesty International, United States of America: the threat of a bad example [AMR 51/114/2003] Aug. 19, 2003, 12.

79. Army Inspector General in Greenberg and Dratel, 709.

80. Surgeon General, 20-12.

81. Dinenna DW. Multiple e-mails. Oct. 27, 2003, Taguba Annex 59.

82. Army Inspector General in Greenberg and Dratel, 710.

83. Arrison J. Sworn statement. Feb. 10, 2004, Taguba Annex 76:12–13.

84. Yee, 143.

85. Army Inspector General in Greenberg and Dratel, 707.

86. Peel M. Hunger strikes. British Medical Journal 1997; 315(7112):829–30.

87. Reyes H. Medical and ethical aspects of hunger strikes in custody and the issue of torture. In *Research in Legal Medicine* (Lübeck: Verlag Schidt-Romhild, 1998), on website of International Committee of the Red Cross, http://www.icrc.org/Web/Eng/siteeng0.nsf/iwpList74/F18AA3CE47E5A98C1256B66005D6E29.

88. Silove D, Curtis J, Mason C, et al. Ethical considerations in the management of asylum seekers on hunger strike. JAMA 1996; 276:410–15.

89. Brockman B. Food refusal in prisoners: a communication or a method of self-killing? The role of the psychiatrist and resulting ethical challenges. Journal of Medical Ethics 1999;25:451–56.

90. Greenberg JK. Hunger striking: the constitutionality of force-feeding. Fordham Law Review 1983;51:747–70.

91. Sunshine SC. Should a hunger-striking prisoner be allowed to die? Boston College Law Review 1984;25:423–58.

92. Ansbacher R. Force feeding hunger strikers: a framework for analysis. University of Florida Law Review 1983;35:99–129.

93. Reyes H. Medical and ethical aspects of hunger strikes in custody and the issue of torture. In *Research in Legal Medicine* (Lübeck: Verlag Schidt-Romhild, 1998), on website of International Committee of Red Cross, http://www.icrc.org/Web/Eng/siteeng0.nsf/iwpList74/F18AA3CE47E5A98BC1256B66005D6E29.

94. Oguz YN, Miles SH. The physician and prison hunger strikes: reflections on the experience in Turkey. Journal of Medical Ethics 2005;31:169–72.

95. 12th Military Policy Detachment. CID Report of Investigation-Final-Supplemental-0140-03-CID259-61190-5H9A (Dham Spah, Deceased). Jan. 24, 2004, unpaginated.

96. Armed Forces Institute of Pathology. Autopsy ME03-368 and death certificate. Aug. 25, 2003. MEDCOM 71–76, 189.

97. 22nd Military Policy Battalion. CID Report of Investigation-Final-Supplemental-0136-03-CID259-61187-5H9A (Najem Mohamed Abed). Jun. 4, 2004, unpaginated.

98. Armed Forces Institute of Pathology. Autopsy ME03-386 and death certificate. Aug. 24, 2003. MEDCOM 81–84, 187.

99. Wallin N. Sworn statement. Jan. 26, 2004, in Greenberg and Dratel, 472.

100. Melone R. Sworn statement. (File #: 0134002 CID 369-23533). Mar. 2, 2004, unpaginated.

101. Guantanamo hunger strikers double. BBC News Dec. 30, 2005.

102. Lewis NA. Guantánamo prisoners go on hunger strike. New York Times Sep. 18, 2005.

103. Gall C. Tales of despair from Guantánamo. New York Times Jun. 17, 2003.

104. Okie S. Glimpses of Guantanamo—medical ethics and the war on terror. New England Journal of Medicine 2005;353:2529–34.

105. Golden T. Tough U.S. steps in hunger strike at camp in Cuba. New York Times Feb. 9, 2006.

106. Amnesty International. Iraq: Memorandum on Concerns Relating to Law and Order [MDE 14/157/2003] Jul. 23, 2003, 3.

107. [Name redacted]. IG [Inspector General] Report of Army Detainee Operations Inspection. Aug. 18, 2004, MEDCOM 403.

108. Army Inspector General in Greenberg and Dratel, 710–11.

109. Army Regulation 190-8: Enemy Prisoners of War, Retained Personnel, Civilian Internees and Other Detainees. Oct. 1, 1997.

110. Army Regulation 40-5: Preventive Medicine. Oct. 15, 1990.

111. [Name redacted]. Preventive medicine at EPW and Incarceration Facilities. Nov. 7, 2003, MEDCOM 394–98.

112. Army Inspector General in Greenberg and Dratel, 705–713.

113. Karpinski J. Deposition. Jul. 18, 2004, DOD 000089.

114. Army Inspector General in Greenberg and Dratel, 660.

115. Army Inspector General in Greenberg and Dratel, 707, 710.

116. Army Inspector General in Greenberg and Dratel, 708.

117. [Name redacted]. Preventive medicine at EPW and Incarceration Facilities. Nov. 5, 2003, MEDCOM 398–99.

118. Investigation of Riot at Camp Cropper. Jun. 9, 2003, Taguba Annex 5.

119. ICRC in Greenberg and Dratel, 399.

120. US Army 40th Military Police Battalion. Escape and Shooting at Abu Gharaib [sic]. Jun. 21, 2003, Taguba Annex 7.

121. Army Inspector General in Greenberg and Dratel, 635, 648.

122. Fay in Greenberg and Dratel, 1042.

123. Pappas T. Sworn statement. May 14, 2004, DOD 000623.

124. Incident and SPOT [on-the-spot intelligence brief] Reports. Numerous dates, Taguba Annex 103.

125. Fisk R. Saddam's vilest prison has been swept clean, but questions remain. The Independent Sep. 17, 2003.

126. ICRC in Greenberg and Dratel, 403.

127. Fay in Greenberg and Dratel, 1042.

128. Army Inspector General in Greenberg and Dratel, 659.

129. Army Inspector General in Greenberg and Dratel, 661, 707.

130. Abu Ghraib in a nutshell, recent activity. Undated [from 2003–2004], Taguba Annex 40.

131. Joint Interrogation & Detention Center Briefing Slides. Abu Ghurayb. Undated [from 2003–2004], Taguba Annex 40.

132. Army Inspector General in Greenberg and Dratel 635, 658.

133. Global Security. Abu Ghurayb Prison. Global Security.com May 23, 2005.

134. US detainee death toll hits 108. BBC News Apr. 28, 2005.

135. Mraz S. Landstuhl nurse treated the "real bad guys" during time in Iraq. Stars and Stripes (European edition) Dec. 19, 2005.

136. Winkenwerder W, Kiley KC, Arthur DC, et al. Doctors and torture. New England Journal of Medicine 2005;351:1572–73.

137. Surgeon General.

138. Bloche MG, Marks JH. When doctors go to war. New England Journal of Medicine 2004;352:3–6.

139. Surgeon General, 7-1-6.

140. Surgeon General, 7-1.

141. Physicians for Human Rights. Break them down: systematic use of psychological torture by US Forces, 2005.

142. Working Group, 31–32.

143. American Forces Information Service. Guantanamo Detainees Receiving "First-Rate" Medical Care. Feb. 18, 2005.

144. Saar and Viveca, 67.

145. ICRC in Greenberg and Dratel, 388.

146. Fay in Greenberg and Dratel, 1042.

147. Surgeon General, 20-7.

148. Surgeon General, 20-7.

149. Church, 19–21.

150. Army Inspector General in Greenberg and Dratel, 731.

CHAPTER 6: SILENCE

1. Al-Zayiadi HMM, Detainee #19446, 1242. Statement to Taguba investigators. Jan. 18, 2004, in Greenberg and Dratel, 501.

2. Hiadar Sabar Abed Miktub Al-Aboodi, Detainee #13077. Statement to Taguba investigators. Jan. 20, 2004, in Greenberg and Dratel, 488.

3. Sivits J. Sworn statement. Jan. 14, 2004, Taguba Annex 25/26.

4. England L. Sworn statement. Jan. 14, 2004, Taguba Annex 25/26.

5. Harmon S. Sworn statement. Jan. 14–15, 2004, Taguba Annex 25/26.

6. Wisdom MC. Sworn statement. Jan. 15, 2004, Taguba 25/26.

7. Sivits J. Sworn statement. Jan. 14, 2004, Taguba Annex 25/26.

8. England L. Sworn statement. Jan. 15, 2004, Taguba Annex 25/26.

9. Fay in Greenberg and Dratel, 1079.

10. Langianese S. Sworn statement. Jan. 20, 2004, in Greenberg and Dratel, 490.

11. Porter C. Sworn statement. Jan. 20, 2004, in Greenberg and Dratel, 490.

12. Spencer L. Sworn statement. Jan. 21, 2004, in Greenberg and Dratel, 477.

13. Oppel RA. Sergeant in Abu Ghraib case pleads guilty to 8 counts. New York Times Oct. 21, 2004.

14. Potter B. Reservist pleads guilty in prison scandal. USA Today Oct. 20, 2004.

15. Sivits J. Sworn statement. Jan. 14, 2004, Taguba Annex 25/26.

16. Wisdom MC. Sworn statement. Jan. 15, 2004, Taguba Annex 25/26.

17. Sivits J. Sworn statement. Jan. 14, 2004, Taguba Annex 25/26.

18. England L. Sworn statement. Jan. 15, 2004, Taguba Annex 25/26.

19. Sivits J. Sworn statement. Jan. 14, 2004, Taguba Annex 25/26.

20. England L. Sworn statement. Jan. 15, 2004, Taguba Annex 25/26.

21. Harmon S. Sworn statement. Jan. 14–15, 2004, Taguba Annex 25/26.

22. England L. Sworn statement. Jan. 15, 2004, Taguba Annex 25/26.

23. Sivits J. Sworn statement. Jan. 14, 2004, Taguba Annex 25/26.

24. Fuoco M, Lash C. Abuse no secret to many in Iraq. Pittsburgh Post-Gazette Jun. 27, 2004.

25. Gibson G. Other abuses at prison recounted. Baltimore Sun Aug. 6, 2004.

26. Zernicke K. Only a few spoke up on abuse as many soldiers stayed silent. New York Times May 22, 2004.

27. 3rd Military Police Group, 78th Military Police Detachment. CID Report of Investigation-Final C/SSI-0124-04-CID259-80199-/5C1Q2/5Y2E. Jul. 5, 2004, DODDOACID 004821–33.

28. Fay in Greenberg and Dratel 1079, 1122.

29. Surgeon General, 20-9.

30. Nelson H. Psychological Assessment. [Undated 2004] Taguba Annex 1 in Greenberg and Dratel, 448–50.

31. Mortenson D. Medic says Pittman hit, slapped inmates. North County Times (Calif.) Aug. 31, 2004.

32. Wallin N. Sworn statement. Jan. 26, 2004, in Greenberg and Dratel, 472–3.

33. US Naval Criminal Investigation Services. Investigative action. Oct. 8, 2003, 3545.

34. Layton R. Sworn statement. Jan. 14, 2004, Taguba Annex 25/26.

35. Layton R. Sworn statement. Jan. 14, 2004, Taguba Annex 25/26.

36. Wallin N. Sworn statement. Jan. 26, 2004, in Greenberg and Dratel, 472–73.

37. Cavallaro A. Sworn testimony. Feb. 15, 2004, Taguba Annex 61, 53.

38. Clinical record from Abu Ghraib. Mar. 16, 2004, MEDCOM 623–44.

39. ICRC in Greenberg and Dratel, 390–91.

40. Fisher I. Searing uncertainty for Iraqis missing loved ones. New York Times Jun. 1, 2004.

41. US Army 3rd Military Police Group, 78th Military Police Detachment. Final C/SSI-0180-04-CID259-80227-/5C1C/5Y2E/5X1. Aug. 5, 2004, DODDOACID 005090–5132.

42. Human Rights Watch. Leadership failure: firsthand accounts of torture of Iraqi detainees by the US Army 82nd Airborne Division. 2005;17:3(G).

43. Army, Office of the Staff Judge Advocate. AR 15-6 Investigation in the broken jaw injury of [Censored]. Dec. 31, 2003. 001198–269.

44. Marshall A. US troops tortured Iraqis in Mosul, documents show. Reuters Mar. 26, 2005.

45. Emergency Care and Treatment Clinical Note. [Date redacted], 001214.

46. [Name redacted, of 6th Company, 526 FSB]. Sworn statement. Dec. 16, 2003, 1239.

47. [Name redacted, of unit redacted]. Sworn statement. Dec. 28, 2003, 1243.

48. [Name redacted, of unit redacted]. Sworn statement. Dec. 24, 2003, 1241.

49. [6th Company, 526 FSB]. Sworn statement. Dec. 16, 2003, 001239.

50. Army 3rd Military Police Group, 78th Military Police Detachment. CID Report of Investigation Initial/Final SSI-0234-04-CID259-80271-/5C2/5Y2E/5X1. Aug. 2, 2004, DODDOACID 005245–48.

51. Army 3rd Military Police Group, 78th Military Police Detachment. CID report of Investigation-Final-0189-04-CID259-80233-/5C2B/5Y2E /5X1/5M3A. Jul. 20, 2004, DODDOACID 000545–49.

52. 48th Military Police Detachment, 3rd Military Police Group. CID Report of Investigation-Final/Supplemental/SSI-0213-2004-CID259-80250-/5C2B/5Y2E. Jun. 17, 2005, DOD 044418–96.

53. 11th Military Police Battalion, 6th Military Police Group. Operation Review of CID Report of Investigation (0174-03-CID469-60225). May 19, 2004, DODDOACID 005993–6020.

54. 3rd Military Police Group, 78th Military Police Detachment. CID Report of Investigation-Final C/SSI-0147-04-CID259-80210-/5C1R2/5Y2E /5X1. Jul. 17, 2004, DODDOACID-005015–5040.

55. Strategic Air Command, 78th Military Police Detachment. CID Report 3rd status/SSI-0106-04-CID259-80185-/5C1Q2/5Y2E/6F8A/6C1/5H9B/5M3. Jun. 22, 2004, DODDOACID 005544–561.

56. Lannen S. Soldier: Guantanamo MPs beat me. Lexington Herald-Leader (Ky.) May 26, 2004.

57. GI attacked during training. CBS News Nov. 3, 2004.

58. Kristof ND. Beating Specialist Baker. New York Times Jun. 5, 2004.

59. Army 43rd Military Police Detachment, 10th Military Police Battalion. CID Report of Investigation, Final C-0174-03-CID469-60225-/5C1L /5Y2. Feb 5, 2004, DODDOACID 005901–5981.

60. Clinical Record. Jun. 29, 2003, MEDCOM 553–54.

61. Army, 101st Airborne Division. Criminal Investigation. Jan. 14, 2004, 001164–279.

62. US Army 3rd Military Police Group, 78th Military Police Detachment. CID Report of Investigation, Final C/SSI-0180-04-CID259-80227-/5C1C/5Y2E/5X1. Jul. 28, 2004, DODDOACID 001248–65.

63. Debriefer/Interrogator to Chief. Witnessing of harsh treatment to Iraqi detainees held in camp Na'ma. May 8, 2004, DODDOACID 009145–46.

64. A——— S, Detainee # 150422, 1630. Statement. Jan. 17, 2004, in Greenberg and Dratel, 508.

65. Nakhla A. Statement. Jan. 18, 2004, Taguba Annex 25/26.

66. Mustafa JM, Detainee # 150422, 1610. Statement. Jan. 17, 2004, in Greenberg and Dratel, 511.

67. Fay in Greenberg and Dratel, 1082.

68. Zernike K. Ringleader in Iraqi prisoner abuse is sentenced to 10 years. New York Times Feb. 16, 2005.

69. Zernike K. Army reservist's defense rests in Abu Ghraib abuse case. New York Times Jan. 14, 2005.

70. Surgeon General, 20-7.

71. Fay in Greenberg and Dratel, 1121.

72. Surgeon General, 20-7.

73. Mayer J. The experiment. The New Yorker Jul. 11, 2005, 60–71.

74. Hoyt R. Readers' responses to the webcast video editorial entitled "Was there physician complicity in state-sponsored human torture in Guantanamo, Iraq, and Afghanistan?" MedScape 2004;6(4) [posted Oct. 8, 2004].

75. Savage C. Abuse outraged Navy at Guantanamo Bay. International Herald Tribune Mar. 17, 2005.

76. Rana G (International Committee of the Red Cross). The ICRC privilege not to testify: confidentiality in action. Feb. 28, 2004.

77. Department of Defense, Joint Task Force 170, Guantánamo Bay. Various minutes Apr. 10, 2002, to Sep. 23, 2003, DOD 000906–948.

78. ICRC in Greenberg and Dratel, 383–404.

79. ICRC in Greenberg and Dratel, 404.

80. ICRC in Greenberg and Dratel, 384–85.

81. Fay in Greenberg and Dratel, 1066–1070, 1113.

82. Wilkerson J, Carrell D. The American medical PACs' strategy of giving in U.S. House races. Journal of Health Politics, Policy, and Law 1999;24:335–55.

83. Doherty RB. Why the College voiced its concerns on prison abuse. ACP Observer Jul. 2004.

84. Peck P. AMA asks Bush for Iraq prison inquiry. UPI Jun. 14, 2004.

85. Mayor S. AMA calls for inquiry into doctors' role in abuse of prisoners. BMJ 2004;329:993.

86. Lifton RJ. Doctors and torture. New England Journal of Medicine 2004;351:415–16.

87. Miles SH. Abu Ghraib: Its legacy for military medicine. Lancet 2004;364:725–29.

88. Mayor S. Medical bodies urge investigation of alleged involvement in torture. BMJ 2004;329:473.

89. American Medical Association, Council on Ethical and Judicial Affairs. Opinion E-2.067 Torture (I, III). Dec. 1999.

90. Robeznieks A. Military doctors reminded of wartime roles. AMEDNEWS.com Sep. 27, 2004.

91. Murphy T, Johnson PJ. Torture and human rights. AMA Virtual Mentor Jun. 8, 2005.

92. Rubenstein L, Pross C, Davidoff F, et al. Coercive US interrogation policies: a challenge to medical ethics. JAMA 2005;294:1544–49.

93. McCain J. McCain statement on detainee amendments. (Press release.) Oct. 5, 2005.

94. American Psychiatric Association. Statement on Psychiatric Practices at Guantanamo Bay. Jun. 27, 2005.

95. American Psychological Association. Report of Presidential Task Force on Psychological Ethics and National Security. June 2005.

96. Wilks M. A stain on medical ethics. Lancet 2005;366:429–31.

97. Behnke S, Wilks M, Lifton RJ, et al. Psychological warfare? A debate on the role of mental health professionals in military interrogations at Guantanamo, Abu Ghraib and beyond. (Radio transcript). Democracy Now! Aug. 11, 2005.

98. Rubenstein L (Physicians for Human Rights). Letter responding to the American Psychological Association's recommendations on torture and national security. Jul. 15, 2005.

99. McKelvey T. First, do some harm. American Prospect Aug. 31, 2001.

100. Lewis NA. Guantánamo tour focuses on medical ethics. New York Times Nov. 13, 2005.

101. Ex-CIA chief: Cheney "VP for torture." CNN Nov. 18, 2005.

102. American College of Physicians. Open Letter to John McCain. Sep. 21, 2005.

103. Maves MD (CEO, American Medical Association). Letter to members of United States Senate Committee on Appropriations. Nov. 1, 2005.

104. American Psychological Association. Action Alert: Support the McCain Amendment calling for prohibition on cruel, inhuman, or degrading treatment of U.S. detainees. Oct. 2005.

105. Peck P. AMA to examine ethics of physician involvement in prisoner interrogations. MedPage Today Nov. 8, 2005.

106. American Public Health Association. Condemning the cooperation of health professional personnel in physical and mental abuse and torture of military prisoners and detainees. (Press release.) Nov. 9, 2004.

107. Office of the Chief Army Nurse Corps to American Nurses Association. (Letter.) Feb. 24, 2005.

108. Board, American Society for Bioethics and Humanities. Letter to President Bush. Aug. 2, 2004.

109. Lee B. The stain of torture. Washington Post Jul. 1, 2005, A25.

110. Physicians for Human Rights. The U.S. health professionals' call to prevent torture and abuse of detainees in U.S. custody. 2005.

111. World Medical Association. Physicians' ethical duty in times of armed conflict reiterated. (Press release.) Oct. 10, 2004.

112. World Medical Association. Physicians should report acts of torture, says WMA president. (Press release.) June 12, 2004.

113. Fay in Greenberg and Dratel, 1121–22.

114. Army Inspector General in Greenberg and Dratel, 777.

115. Gilmore GJ. Medical personnel didn't commit widespread detainee abuse, says DoD. Armed Forces Information Service Feb. 11, 2005.

116. Church, 20.

117. Surgeon General, 1-4-6, 14-1.

118. Surgeon General, 14-1.

119. Army Criminal Investigation Command. Sworn statement of Robert Melone. (File # 0134002 CID-369-23533). Aug. 5, 2004, unpaginated.

120. [Name and unit redacted, Kandahar, Afghanistan]. Feb. 11, 2002, DOD 043624–25.

121. [Name and unit redacted, Kandahar, Afghanistan]. Feb. 16, 2002, DOD 043636.

122. Surgeon General, 16-1.

123. Army Regulation 15-6: Final report. Investigation into FBI allegations of detainee abuse at Guantanamo Bay, Cuba Detention Facility. Apr. 1, 2005 (amended Jun. 9, 2005).

124. Extensive FBI e-mails protesting Army abuse are posted at http://www.aclu.org/torturefoia/. Documents released throughout 2004, May 2005, Jun. 2005.

125. Surgeon General, 15-1.

126. Multiple clinical records, MEDCOM 645–759. ACLU documents released May, Jun. 2005.

127. Surgeon General, 16-2.

128. Surgeon General, 17-2-3.

129. Galvin R. The complex world of military medicine: a conversation with William Winkenwerder. Health Affairs Aug. 4, 2005 (Web exclusive).

130. Fay in Greenberg and Dratel, 1071.

131. Jacoby LE, USN Director, Defense Intelligence Agency to Undersecretary of Defense for Intelligence. Alleged detainee abuse by TF-62 personnel. Jun. 25, 2004, 02596–97.

132. Bloche MG, Marks JH. When doctors go to war. New England Journal of Medicine 2004;352:3–6.

133. Shane S. Republicans help whistleblowers. New York Times Feb. 17, 2006.

134. US Naval Criminal Investigation Service. Investigative Action, Whidbey Island—Navy Hospital Oak Harbor alleged assault of Iraqi prisoners of war. Oct. 8, 2003, 3545.

135. Army Criminal Investigation Service. Abu Ghraib investigation May 13, 2004, DOD 880.

136. Lewis, N. Red Cross finds detainee abuse in Guantánamo. New York Times. Nov. 20, 2004.

137. British Medical Association. Recommendations from *The Medical Profession and Human Rights: Handbook for a Changing Agenda*. London, 2001.

138. International Dual Loyalty Working Group (Physicians for Human Rights and School of Public Health and Primary Health Care, University of Cape Town, Health Sciences Faculty). Dual Loyalty and Human Rights in Health Professional Practice; Proposed Guidelines and Institutional Mechanisms. 2002.

139. International Committee of the Red Cross. How visits by the ICRC can help prisoners cope with the effects of traumatic stress. Jan. 1, 1996.

PART III: "PLAIN LANGUAGE"

CHAPTER 7: GRAVE BREACHES

1. Title 18, Part I, Chapter 118 § 2441.

2. Yoo J, Delabunty RJ. Application of treaties and laws to al Qaeda and Taliban detainees. Jan. 9, 2002, in Greenberg and Dratel, 38–79.

3. Bybee JS. Application of treaties and laws to Al Qaeda and Taliban detainees. Jan. 22, 2002, in Greenberg and Dratel, 81–117.

4. Bybee JS. Status of Taliban forces under Article 4 of the Third Geneva Convention of 1949. Feb. 7, 2002, in Greenberg and Dratel, 136–43.

5. Cole D. What Bush wants to hear. New York Review of Books 2005; 52(18).

6. Secretary of Defense. Status of Taliban and Al Qaida. Jan. 19, 2002, in Greenberg and Dratel, 80.

7. Powell C. Draft decision memorandum for the president on the applicability of the Geneva Convention to the conflict in Afghanistan. [undated] in Greenberg and Dratel, 122–25.

8. Taft WH IV. Comments on your paper on the Geneva Convention. Feb. 2, 2002, in Greenberg and Dratel, 129–33.

9. Ashcroft J. Dear Mr. President. Feb. 1, 2002, in Greenberg and Dratel, 126–27.

10. Gonzales AR. Decisions re application of the Geneva Convention on prisoners of war to the conflict with Al Qaeda and the Taliban. Jan. 25, 2002, in Greenberg and Dratel, 118–21.

11. Bush G. Humane treatment of al Qaeda and Taliban detainees. Feb. 7, 2002, in Greenberg and Dratel, 134–35.

12. Yee, 47–48.

13. Bybee JS. Application of treaties and laws to Al Qaeda and Taliban detainees. Jan. 22, 2002, in Greenberg and Dratel, 85.

14. Bybee JS. Application of treaties and laws to Al Qaeda and Taliban detainees. Jan. 22, 2002, in Greenberg and Dratel, 108.

15. U.S.C. 18: PART I; 113C — Torture.

16. Bybee JS. Potential legal constraints applicable to interrogations of persons captured by US Armed Forces in Afghanistan. Feb. 26, 2002, in Greenberg and Dratel, 144–71.

17. Bybee JS. Standards of Conduct for Interrogation Under 18 USC. 2340-2340A. Aug. 1, 2002, in Greenberg and Dratel, 172–217.

18. Phifer J. Request for Approval of Counter Resistance Strategies. Oct. 11, 2002, in Greenberg and Dratel, 227–28.

19. DunLeavey ME. Counter Resistance Strategies. Oct. 11, 2002, in Greenberg and Dratel, 225.

20. Hill JR. Counter Resistance Techniques. Oct. 25, 2002, in Greenberg and Dratel, 223.

21. Beaver D. Legal brief on proposed counter-resistance strategies. Oct. 11, 2002, in Greenberg and Dratel, 229–35.

22. Rumsfeld D. Counter Resistance Techniques. Nov. 27, 2002, in Greenberg and Dratel, 237.

23. Secretary of Defense. Counter Resistance Techniques. Jan. 15, 2002, in Greenberg and Dratel, 239.

24. Working Group Report. Detainee interrogations in the global war on terrorism. Mar. 6, 2002, in Greenberg and Dratel, 241–85.

25. Working Group Report. Detainee interrogations in the global war on terrorism. Apr. 4, 2003, in Greenberg and Dratel, 286–359.

26. Working Group Report. Detainee interrogations in the global war on terrorism. Apr. 4, 2003, in Greenberg and Dratel, 333–34.

27. Working Group Report. Detainee interrogations in the global war on terrorism. Apr. 4, 2003, in Greenfield and Dratel, 346.

28. Working Group Report. Detainee interrogations in the global war on terrorism. Apr. 4, 2003, in Greenberg and Dratel, 335.

29. Secretary of Defense. Memorandum for the Commander, US Southern Command; Counter Resistance Techniques in the War on Terrorism. Apr. 16, 2003, in Greenberg and Dratel, 360–65.

30. Secretary of Defense. Memorandum for the Commander, US South-

ern Command; Counter Resistance Techniques in the War on Terrorism. Apr. 16, 2003, in Greenberg and Dratel, 360–65.

31. Secretary of Defense. Memorandum for the Commander, US Southern Command; Counter Resistance Techniques in the War on Terrorism. Apr. 16, 2003, in Greenberg and Dratel, 364.

32. Secretary of Defense. Memorandum for the Commander, US Southern Command; Counter Resistance Techniques in the War on Terrorism. Apr. 16, 2003, in Greenberg and Dratel, 363.

33. Secretary of Defense. Memorandum for the Commander, US Southern Command; Counter Resistance Techniques in the War on Terrorism. Apr. 16, 2003, in Greenberg and Dratel, 364.

34. Secretary of Defense. Memorandum for the Commander, US Southern Command; Counter Resistance Techniques in the War on Terrorism. Apr. 16, 2003, in Greenberg and Dratel, 364.

35. Fay in Greenberg and Dratel, 1037–38.

36. Joint Interrogation and Debriefing Center. Interrogation Rules of Engagement (IROE) Jan. 23, 2004. Taguba Annex 40:26–28.

37. Surgeon General, 18-12.

38. Church, 20.

39. Spannaus E. Congress must take up torture probe. Executive Intelligence Review Sep. 10, 2004.

40. Myers L. Top terrorist hunter's divisive views. NBCtv. Oct. 15, 2003.

41. Sanchez R. Combined Joint Task Forces Interrogation and Counter Resistance Policy. Oct. 12, 2003, in Greenberg and Dratel, 460–65.

42. Fay in Greenberg and Dratel, 1046–1047.

43. Taguba in Greenberg and Dratel, 410.

44. Ryder, Taguba Annex 19.

45. Fay in Greenberg and Dratel, 1030–31.

46. Amnesty International. Foreword, Report 2005. Apr. 2005, London.

47. Bush GW. Detention, treatment and trial of certain non-citizens in the war against terrorism. Nov. 13, 2001, in Greenberg and Dratel, 25–28.

48. Robertson G. *Crimes Against Humanity: The Struggle for Global Justice.* New York: The New Press, 1990.

49. Gonzales AR. Decisions re application of the Geneva Convention on prisoners of war to the conflict with Al Qaeda and the Taliban. Jan. 25, 2002, in Greenberg and Dratel, 119.

50. UNESCO Committee on the Theoretical Basis of Human Rights. *Final Report on Human Rights: Comments and Interpretations.* New York: Wingate Press, 1949, 258–59.

51. Donnelly J. *International Human Rights.* San Francisco: Westview Press, 1993.

52. Zakaria F. Psst . . . no one loves a torturer. Newsweek Nov. 14, 2005.

53. Priest D. CIA puts harsh tactics on hold. Washington Post Apr. 27, 2004, A1.

54. Cole D. Torture makes justice impossible. Los Angeles Times Dec. 3, 2005.

55. Bureau of Democracy, Human Rights, and Labor, United States State Department. Country Reports on Human Rights Practices: China— 2004. Feb. 28, 2005.

56. Cody E. Citing Abu Ghraib, China rejects U.S. on rights; Washington has no business judging others, Beijing says. Washington Post Mar. 4, 2005.

57. Parliament of Europe. Resolution 1433 (2005) Lawfulness of detentions by the United States in Guantánamo Bay. Apr. 26, 2005, http://assembly.coe .int/Main.asp?link=http://assembly.coe.int/documents/adoptedtext/ ta05/ERES1433.htm.

58. Lindsay D. German prosecutor won't pursue Rumsfeld case. Der Spiegel Feb. 10, 2005.

59. Aldinger C. Rumsfeld debating whether to avoid Germany. Reuters Feb. 4, 2005.

60. Belgium to curb war crimes law. BBC News Jun. 23, 2003.

61. Assistant Secretary of Defense. Medical Program Principles and Procedures for the Protection and Treatment of Detainees in the Custody of the Armed Forces of the United States. Jun. 3, 2005.

62. Rhem KT. DoD issues guidance for medical personnel dealing with detainees. Armed Forces Information Service Jun. 16, 2005.

63. Kiley KC. Approval of findings and recommendations of functional assessment team concerning detainee medical operations for OEF, GTMO, and OIF. May 24, 2005, unpaginated letter appended to Surgeon General report.

CHAPTER 8: WHY OPPOSE TORTURE?

1. Lifton 1973.

2. Lifton 1973, 104.

3. Simerman J. East Bay soldiers back up rationale. Contra Costa (Calif.) Times. May 9, 2004, A1.

4. Ruthven M. *Torture: The Grand Conspiracy.* London: Weidenfeld and Nicolson, 1978, 281–98.

5. Froomkin D. Cheney's "dark side" is showing. Washington Post Nov. 7, 2005.

6. Lincoln A. Letter to Charles Drake and Others. In *Lincoln: Speeches and Writings*, vol. 2 (New York: Library of America, 1999), 523.

7. Bush G. Memorandum for the Vice President et al. Humane Treatment of al Qaeda and Taliban detainees, in Greenberg and Dratel, 134–35.

8. George Bush. News conference. Nov. 5, 2001.

9. Proctor R. *Racial Hygiene: Medicine Under the Nazis.* Cambridge, Mass.: Harvard University Press, 1992.

10. Muller-Hill B. *Murderous Science.* New York: Oxford University Press, 1988.

11. Block S, Reddaway P. Psychiatrists and dissenters in the Soviet Union, in Stover and Nightingale, 132–63.

12. Koryagin A. Unwilling patients. Lancet 1981;1(8224):821–24.

13. Darby J. Sworn statement. Jan. 14, 2004, Taguba Annex 25/26.

14. Hathaway OA. The promise and limits of the international law of torture, in *Torture: A Collection*, ed. Levinson S. (New York: Oxford University Press, 2004), 199–212.

15. Army Inspector General in Greenberg and Dratel, 630–907.

16. Fay in Greenberg and Dratel, 1018–1131.

17. Church.

18. Surgeon General.

19. British Medical Association, 1.

20. Wiesel E. Without conscience. New England Journal of Medicine 2005;352:1511–13.

21. Miles SH. *The Hippocratic Oath and the Ethics of Medicine* (New York: Oxford University Press, 2004), ix.

22. Von Staden H. "In a pure and holy way": personal and professional conduct in the Hippocratic Oath. Journal of the History of Medicine and Allied Sciences 1996;51:406–408.

APPENDIX 1: INTERROGATING **GTMO** 063:

CASE AND DISCUSSION GUIDE

1. ORCON [Authoring agency classified by Originator Control]. Interrogation Log Detainee 063. http://www1.umn.edu/humanrts/OathBetrayed/inter-log-det-063.pdf. (Accessed Oct. 23, 2008.)

2. Zagorin A, Duffy M. Inside the interrogation of detainee 063. Time Jun. 20, 2005, pp. 26–33.

3. Department of Defense. Guantanamo provides valuable intelligence information. News Release 592–05. Jun. 12, 2005.

4. United States Army. Final Report Investigation into FBI Allegations of Detainee Abuse at Guantanamo Bay, Cuba Detention Facility [section titled "First Special Interrogation Plan," pp. 13–21]. Jun. 5, 2005. http://www1.umn.edu/humanrts/OathBetrayed/d20050714report.pdf. (Accessed Oct. 23, 2008.)

5. AR 15–6 Report, GTMO Investigation, FBI Allegations of Abuse [assorted documents of various dates]. http://www1.umn.edu/humanrts/OathBetrayed/Schmidt-Furlow%20Report%20Enclosures%20I.pdf. (Accessed Oct. 23, 2008.)

6. AR 15–6 Report, GTMO Investigation, FBI Allegations of Abuse [assorted interviews of various dates]. http://www1.umn.edu/humanrts/OathBetrayed/Schmidt-Furlow%20Report%20Enclosures%20II.pdf. (Accessed Oct. 23, 2008.)

7. Bashour TT, Gualberto A, Ryan C. Atrioventricular block in accidental hypothermia—a case report. Angiology 1989;40:63–66.

8. Church A. Untitled Report for Secretary of Defense. Mar. 2005. http://www.aclu.org/pdfs/safefree/church_353365_20080430.pdf. (Accessed Oct. 23, 2008.)

9. Mayer J. The Dark Side. New York: Doubleday Press, 2008.

10. Letter from Michael Gelles. Posted on Psyche, Science and Society. http://psychoanalystsopposewar.org/blog/2007/03/21/whistle-blower

-michael-gelles-throws-in-lot-with-pro-abuse-american-psychological
-association/. (Accessed Oct. 23, 2008.)

11. United States Army. FM 34–52. Intelligence Interrogation. Washington,
DC, Dec. 28, 1992, pp. 61–69. http://www.loc.gov/rr/frd/Military_Law/
pdf/intel_interrogation_sept-1992.pdf. (Accessed Oct. 23, 2008.)

12. Moreno J. *Mind Wars: Brain Research and National Defense*, pp. 61–82.
Washington, DC: Dana Press, 2006.

13. CIA. KUBARK Counterintelligence Interrogation. Jul. 1963. Section
IX: H. http://www.gwu.edu/~nsarchiv/NSAEBB/NSAEBB27/01–01.htm.
(Accessed Oct. 23, 2008.)

14. The Intelligence Science Board. Educing Information Interrogation:
Science and Art. National Defense Intelligence University. 2006. http://
www1.umn.edu/humanrts/OathBetrayed/Intelligence%20Science
%20Board%202006.pdf. (Accessed Oct. 23, 2008.)

15. *Trials of War Criminals before the Nuremberg Military Tribunals. Nuremberg Code: Directives for Human Experimentation*, pp. 181–82. Washington, DC: U.S. Government Printing Office, 1949. http://ohsr.od.nih
.gov/guidelines/nuremberg.html. (Accessed Oct. 23, 2008.)

16. Annas GJ. *American Bioethics: Crossing Human Rights and Health Law
Boundaries*, pp. 159–66. Oxford: Oxford University Press, 2005.

17. United Nations. Convention against Torture and Other Cruel, Inhuman or Degrading Treatment or Punishment 39/46. 1984. http://www
.unhchr.ch/html/menu3/b/h_cat39.htm. (Accessed Oct. 23, 2008.)

18. United Nations. Body of Principles for the Protection of All Persons
under Any Form of Detention or Imprisonment. 1988. http://www
.unhchr.ch/html/menu3/b/h_comp36.htm. (Accessed Oct. 23, 2008.)

19. Geneva Convention Relative to the Treatment of Prisoners of War.
Aug. 12, 1949. http://www.unhchr.ch/html/menu3/b/91.htm. (Accessed
Oct. 23, 2008.)

20. United Nations. Principles of Medical Ethics Relevant to the Role of
Health Personnel, Particularly Physicians, in the Protection of Prisoners
and Detainees Against Torture and Other Cruel, Inhuman or Degrading Treatment or Punishment (Resolution 37/194). 1982. http://www
.unhchr.ch/html/menu3/b/h_comp40.htm. (Accessed Oct. 23, 2008.)

21. World Medical Association. Guidelines for Medical Doctors Concern-

ing Torture and Other Cruel, Inhuman or Degrading Treatment or Punishment in Relation to Detention and Imprisonment (Declaration of Tokyo). 2006 update. http://www.wma.net/e/policy/c18.htm. (Accessed Oct. 23, 2008.)

22. American Medical Association, Council on Ethical and Judicial Affairs. Physician Participation in Interrogation (Opinion 4-I-06). 2006. http://www.ama-assn.org/ama1/pub/upload/mm/475/cejo4io6.doc. (Accessed Oct. 23, 2008.)

23. American Psychiatric Association. Psychiatric Participation in the Interrogation of Detainees. 2006. http://www.psych.org/Departments/EDU/Library/APAOfficialDocumentsandRelated/PositionStatements/200601.aspx. (Accessed Oct. 23, 2008.)

24. Royal College of Psychiatrists. Resolution Condemning Psychiatric Participation in the Interrogation of Detainees. 2006. http://www.rcpsych.ac.uk/pressparliament/pressreleases2006/pr825.aspx. (Accessed Oct. 23, 2008.)

25. *Nuremberg Military Tribunals. Trials of War Criminals before the Nuremberg Military Tribunals under Control Council Law No. 10*, vol. 2, pp. 181–82. Washington, DC: U.S. Government Printing Office, 1949. http://www.hhs.gov/ohrp/references/nurcode.htm. (Accessed Oct. 18, 2008.)

APPENDIX 2: THE AMERICAN PSYCHOLOGICAL ASSOCIATION AND WAR ON TERROR INTERROGATIONS

1. Mayer J. The experiment. New Yorker Jul. 11, 2005.

2. Eban K. Rorschach and awe. Vanity Fair Jul. 17, 2007. http://www.vanityfair.com/politics/features/2007/07/torture200707?printable = true &currentpage = all. (Accessed Oct. 18, 2008.)

3. United States Senate Committee on Armed Services. Testimony of Daniel Baumgartner Jr. Jun. 17, 2008. http://armed-services.senate.gov/statemnt/2008/June/Baumgartner%2006–17–08.pdf. (Accessed Oct. 18, 2008.)

4. Senate Committee on Armed Services. Statement of Dr. Jerald Ogrisseg. Jun. 17, 2008. http://armed-services.senate.gov/statemnt/2008/June/Ogrisseg%2006–17–08.pdf. (Accessed Oct. 18, 2008.)

5. Physicians for Human Rights. Break Them Down: Systematic Use of Psychological Torture by U.S. Forces. May 2005. http://physiciansfor humanrights.org/library/documents/reports/break-them-down-the.pdf. (Accessed Oct. 13, 2008.)

6. Seligman MEP. *Helplessness: On Depression, Development, and Death.* New York: W. H. Freeman Publishing, 1975.

7. Department of Defense. Behavioral Science Consultation Policy. Oct. 2006. http://wikileaks.org/wiki/Guantanmo_Bay_use_of_psychologists _for_interrogations_2006–2008. (Accessed Oct. 18, 2008.)

8. Mayer J. *The Dark Side.* New York: Doubleday Press, 2008.

9. Seligman M. Former APA president Martin Seligman denies involvement in developing CIA tactics. Jul. 14, 2008. http://psychoanalysts opposewar.org/blog/2008/07/14/former-apa-president-martin-seligman -denies-involvement-in-developing-cia-tactics/. (Accessed Oct. 18, 2008.)

10. Arrigo, Jean Maria. The unofficial records of the American Psychological Association Presidential Task Force on Psychological Ethics and National Security, Jun. 2005. Intelligence Ethics Collection, Hoover Institution Archives, Stanford University, Stanford, CA. 2006.

11. American Psychological Association, Peace Psychology Division 48. PENS Task Force Members. http://www.webster.edu/peacepsychology/ tfpens.html. (Accessed Oct. 18, 2008.)

12. Associated Press. AP confirms top secret "Camp 7" inside Gitmo. Feb. 6, 2008. http://cbs2.com/national/Guantanamo.Bay.gitmo.2.647676.html. (Accessed Oct. 18, 2008.)

13. Holloway JD. Helping with post-conflict readjustment. APA Monitor on Psychology 2004;35(2):32. http://www.apa.org/monitor/feb04/helping .html. (Accessed Oct. 18, 2008.)

14. Behnke S. Ethics and interrogations: Comparing and contrasting the American Psychological, American Medical and American Psychiatric Association positions. APA Monitor on Psychology 2006;37(7). http:// www.apa.org/monitor/julaug06/interrogations.html. (Accessed Oct. 18, 2008.)

15. U.S. Senate Armed Services Committee. The Origins of Aggressive Interrogation Techniques [multiple documents, multiple dates]. http:// levin.senate.gov/newsroom/supporting/2008/Documents.SASC.061708 .pdf. (Accessed Oct. 18, 2008.)

16. Thanawala S. Psychologists scrap interrogation ban. Washington Post Aug. 19, 2007. http://www.washingtonpost.com/wp-dyn/content/article/2007/08/19/AR2007081900189.html. (Accessed Oct. 18, 2008.)

17. Lewis, N. Psychologists preferred for detainees. New York Times Jun. 7, 2006.

18. Withhold APA Dues. http://www.withholdapadues.com/. (Accessed Oct. 18, 2008.)

19. Arrigo JM, Long J. APA denunciation and accommodation of abusive interrogations—A lesson for world psychology. Revista Psicologia: Teoria e Prática 2008;10(1):189–99.

20. Olson B, Soldz S. Positive illusions and the necessity of a bright line forbidding psychologist involvement in detainee interrogations. Analyses of Soc Iss Pub Pol 2007;7:1–10.

21. Soldz S, Olson B. Psychologists, detainee interrogations, and torture: Varying perspectives on nonparticipation. In A. Ojeda (ed.), *The Trauma of Psychological Torture*. Westport, CT: Praeger Press, 2008.

22. American Psychological Association. Reports and Resolution Adopted by the APA. http://www.apa.org/ethics/reportsadopted.html. (Accessed Oct. 13, 2008.)

23. American Psychological Association. Psychology and Interrogations: Statement to Senate Select Common on Intelligence. Sep. 19, 2007. http://intelligence.senate.gov/070925/apa.pdf. (Accessed Oct. 13, 2008.)

24. Psychologists for Social Responsibility. http://www.psysr.org/.

25. Nordic Committee of Psychologists Association. Questions about APA's Stand on Psychologists' Participation in U.S. Military and CIA Interrogations. June 15, 2008. http://ethicalapa.com/files/Torture_Nordic_Psych_Assoc_Letter_to_APA.pdf. (Accessed Oct. 18, 2008.)

26. American Psychoanalytic Association. Torture. 2006. http://apsa.org/aboutapsaa/positionstatements/torture/tabid/468/default.aspx. (Accessed Oct. 18, 2008.)

27. International Psychoanalytical Association. Statement on Torture. 2007. http://internationalpsychoanalysis.net:80/2007/09/11/ipa-statement-on-torture-passed-in-berlin-on-july-2007/. (Accessed Oct. 18, 2008.)

28. Royal College of Psychiatrists. Resolution Condemning Psychiatric Participation in the Interrogation of Detainees. 2006. http://www.rcpsych

.ac.uk/pressparliament/pressreleases2006/pr825.aspx. (Accessed Oct. 18, 2008.)

29. United Kingdom Council for Psychotherapy. UKCP Statement on Torture. 2007. http://www.psychotherapy.org.uk:80/iqs/sid.09842940278 929031509767/UKCP_Statement_on_Torture.html. (Accessed Oct. 18, 2008.)

30. International Rehabilitation Council for Torture Victims (Copenhagen). Letter. Aug. 22, 2008. http://www.psysr.org/about/committees/endtorture/ IRCT.pdf. (Accessed Oct. 18, 2008.)

31. Ethical APA. Referendum. 2008. http://ethicalapa.com/referendumtext .html. (Accessed Oct. 18, 2008.)

32. Department of Defense. Statement on 2008 APA Petition Resolution Ballot. Aug. 14, 2008. http://psychoanalystsopposewar.org:80/blog/2008/ 08/22/defense-department-issues-statement-opposing-apa-referendum -there-are-no-neutrals-there/>http://psychoanalystsopposewar.org :80/blog/2008/08/22/defense-department-issues-statement-opposing -apa-referendum-there-are-no-neutrals-there/. (Accessed Oct. 18, 2008.)

33. McCoy A. A Question of Torture: CIA Interrogation, from the Cold War to the War on Terror. New York: Metropolitan Books, 2006.

34. Murray B. A brief history of RxP. APA Monitor on Psychology 2003;34(9) :66.http://www.apa.org/monitor/oct03/rxp.html (Accessed Oct. 18, 2008.)

35. Getting the candidates on record for science. APA's Science Policy Insider News Oct. 2004. http://www.apa.org/ppo/education/CDP_White paper_Jun07.pdf. (Accessed Oct. 18, 2008.)

36. Advocating on Capitol Hill for Psychological Research at DoD. APA's Science Policy Insider News Jun. 2008. http://www.apa.org/ppo/spin/ 608.html. (Accessed Oct. 13, 2008.)

INDEX

Page numbers in *italics* refer to illustrations, maps, and tables

Ghraib compared with, 48, 143; access to medical records at, 55, 64, 150; American Psychological Association and, 187, 191–92, 195, 196; BSCT at, 54, 56, 150; Camp Delta Standard Operating Procedures, xxii; Council of Europe views on, 157; FBI and, 15, 62, 135; Gelles's reports about, 126, 166, 175–76; Geneva Conventions and, 48, 49, 61, 144–47, 149; grave breaches at, 143–51; as gulag, 152; harsh interrogations implemented at, xiii, xv, 148–50; hunger strikes at, 108–11, 129 (see also force feeding); internal reaction force at, 124; interrogation experiments at, xvii–xviii, 169–70, 176–80, 184–185; medical care denied at, 62; medical monitoring at, 59, 60–61, 169–73; mentally ill at, 103, 104, 105; prison investigations at, xx, 64; Red Cross at, 127, 138; silence about, 126, 129, 134, 137, 138

Guardian, xx

Guatemala, 22, 152, 159

"Guidelines for Medical Doctors Concerning Torture . . . ," 5

Guillotin, Joseph-Ignace, 27, 28

guillotine *(louisette; louison)*, 27, 65

GULAG, 152

Gulag Archipelago, The (Solzhenitsyn), 152

Gumaa, Fahin Ali, 71

Habibullah, Mullah (Habib Ullah), *xv*, 68, 87, 89, 91, 135

Habsburg empire, 25

Halifax gibbet, 27

Hamoodi, Yehiya, 9–10

Harman, Sabrina, 45

Hasson, Hadi Abdul Hussain, 80

Hatab, Nagen Sadoon, 89–90, 92–93

Hathaway, Oona, 167

heart attacks, 76, 82–84, 92, 101, 122

heart damage, 108, 109

heart disease, 69, 109

Helmand Province, 92

Helms, Richard, 14

Helsinki Accords (1975), 32, 195

Henry VI (Shakespeare), 4

Herophilius, 30

Herrington, Stuart, 50

Hersh, Seymour M., xx

"high value" persons, xii, 192

Hill, James T., 148

"Hill, Professor," 86

Hippocrates, 168

Hippocratic Oath, 38, 168

Hitler, Adolf, 6

Hodges, Jerry, 79, 95

Hodges, Michael, 122

Holferty, Jerrod, 44

Holocaust, 165

Holzer, Jenny, 21

homicide, 68–96; at Abu Ghraib, 44–45, 71, 72, 83, 95; death certificates and, x, 45, 69, 70, 71, 73–80, 77, 78, 84–89, 91–96; Defense Department response to, 84–87; of Dilawar, 62, 68–71, 87, 89, 134–35; discussion about, 87–90; medical investigations of, 73–74; misclassified as natural death, 82–84; obstructed investigations and, 79–82; prisoner deaths by, 71–73, 90–96; silence about, 137, 139;

House of Representatives, U.S., 132

Hoyt, Robert, 126

"Human Resource Exploitation Manual" (CIA), 14–15, 16, 18

Human Resources Resource Organization (HumRRO), 187

human rights, xii–xiii; U.S. loss of credibility as advocate of, xxvi, 155–56

Human Rights First, 133

Human Rights Watch, xxi, *xxiv*, 81, 82, 100, 133, 159; Red Cross compared with, 126

humiliation, 8, 61

hunger strikes, xxii, 107–11, 114–15, 129; collective, 108, 110

Husaybah prison, 79

ABOUT THE AUTHOR

STEVEN H. MILES, M.D., a professor of medicine at the University of Minnesota Medical School, Minneapolis, is on the faculty of the Center for Bioethics, and has served as president of the American Association of Bioethics and on the ethics task force for President Clinton's Bioethics Health Care Reform Commission. He is a recognized expert in medical ethics, human rights, and international health care. He is the recipient of the Distinguished Service Award of the American Society of Bioethics and Humanities and has been active in state and national health care reform. He is married and gardens in Minneapolis, Minnesota.

ABOUT THE TYPE

This book was set in Electra, a typeface designed for Linotype by W. A. Dwiggins, the renowned type designer (1880–1956). Electra is a fluid typeface, avoiding the contrasts of thick and thin strokes that are prevalent in most modern typefaces.